birth pain

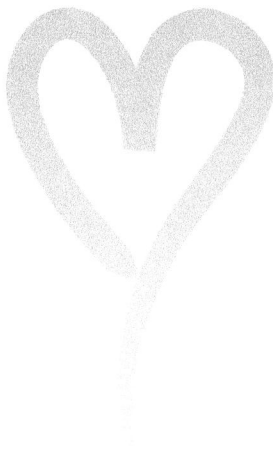

birth pain

POWER TO TRANSFORM!

a guide for pregnant women

Verena Schmid

Fresh ♥ Heart
PUBLISHING

1st British edition

First published in Great Britain in 2011 by
FRESH HEART PUBLISHING
a division of Fresh Heart Ltd
PO Box 225, Chester le Street, DH3 9BQ
www.freshheartpublishing.co.uk

A CIP catalogue record for this publication is available from the British Library

ISBN: 978 1 906619 21 3

The original German text, *Der Geburtsschmerz: Bedeutung und natürliche
Methoden der Schmerzlinderung,* was published by Hippokrates in Stuttgart in
2005. ISBN: 978 3 8304 5309 3. See www.hippokrates.de
Translated from the German by Sylvie Donna
Edited by Sylvie Donna, Trudy Stevens and Shelly Harris-Studdart
Set in Franklin Gothic Book, Bookman Old Style and Bradley Hand ITC
Printed in the UK by Lightning Source UK Ltd
Cover design by Fresh Heart Publishing and Jill Furmanovsky
Cover photo of Aly Neely used with kind permission
Designed and typeset by Fresh Heart Publishing

Disclaimer

While the advice and information contained in this book is believed to be
accurate and true at the time of going to press, neither the author nor the
publisher can accept any legal responsibility for loss, damage or injury
occasioned to any person acting or refraining from action as a result of
information contained herein. These suggestions are guidelines only and
should be used alongside advice from midwives or obstetricians.

Dedication

This book is dedicated to all the women and babies
who taught me through their strength and competence
that birth can be an ecstatic experience.

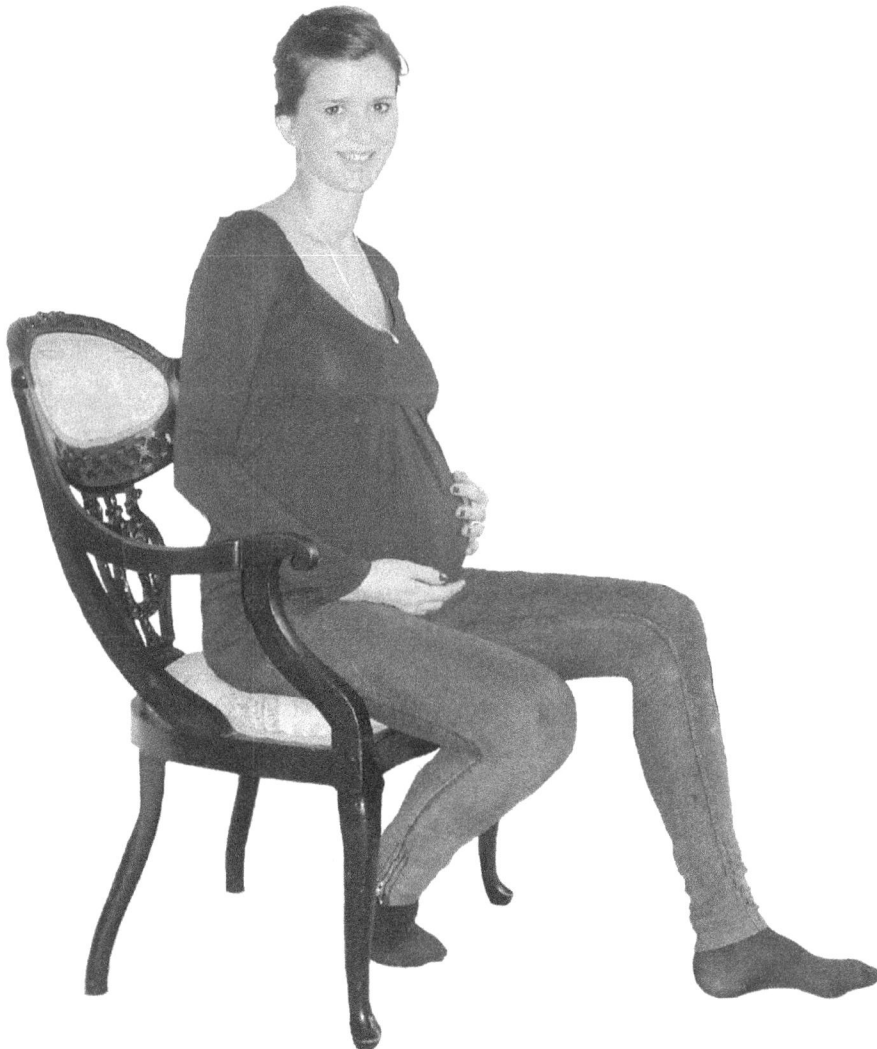

Contents

/ continued overleaf...

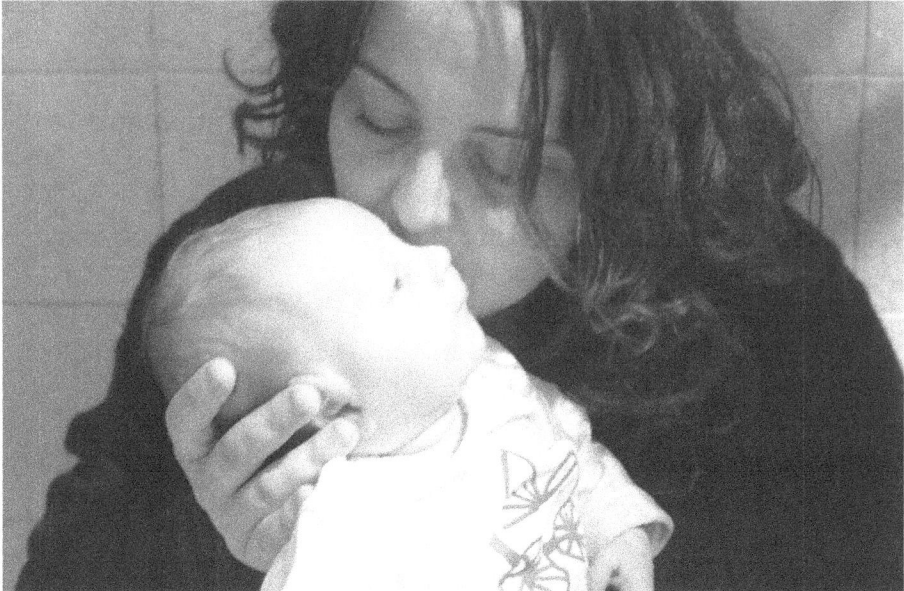

Photo © Sandro Pintus—see www.catpress.org

An overview of issues from the translator and editor...

I find it very understandable that women around 100 years ago were campaigning to have pain relief in childbirth. It also makes sense to me why some women fight hard to *avoid* pain relief now, and also why some women still choose it. But our context for birth is now not what it was 100 years ago.

At the beginning of the 20th century, around 1911, women's lives were very different. There was no birth control beyond withdrawal, abstinence or voluntary celibacy. (Not getting married actually enabled some women to legitimately opt out of the drudgery that marriage and childbearing would often involve.) The work which a married woman would need to do was very physical, tiring and repetitive, and there were only basic cleaning products, materials and equipment (such as a metal bucket and a mop) to make this work possible. When the first baby came along—as all the woman's relatives hoped would happen—a married woman's workload would suddenly increase and it would continue to grow as each subsequent child was added to her household.

In addition, unlike in recent decades, a woman's sexuality was not something which was generally enjoyed, as it often is nowadays. Since men's lives were also usually full of physical hard work for relentless hours in poor conditions (compared to those both men and women enjoy today), a woman's husband would usually return home tired, with little expectation of intimacy but perhaps a great expectation of a quick fumble under the covers, and with no awareness of or interest in anything like a clitoris or a G-spot. Since sex was such a taboo subject and something which often landed women in embarrassing, socially humiliating situations (when they became pregnant outside marriage, for example, or when they contracted some kind of STD), it is unlikely that many women actually enjoyed sex. Given the emotional gulf which must have existed between many sexual partners in those days, it seems more likely that sex was something to be feared... Not only might it be painful and uncomfortable, it might also result in yet another expensive, exhausting unwanted pregnancy, which the family would again not really be able to afford.

Labour and birth must also have been a focus of fear because—before widespread sanitation (as a result of piped water and flushing toilets)—and before the easy availability of affordable or free healthcare (before the NHS was set up in 1947), too many labours ended in either a dead or a sickly mother or baby. And too often, because of certain practices which had become commonplace in hospitals even in the 1920s and 1930s—the routine use of episiotomy and forceps for birth, for example—having a baby would have meant a great deal of pain postnatally for the mother and even more painful sex... Not only would the woman be fearful of another pregnancy, when approached by her husband, she would also be worried about suffering even greater discomfort or injury as a result of poorly healed episiotomies or painful scar tissue, which could not easily be treated. Back-street abortions would have exacerbated many women's pain and they are a further testimony to the negative associations sex must have had for too many women just 100 years ago. A few decades before, in 1853, when Queen Victoria had made the use of anaesthesia for childbirth seem acceptable by using it herself, women must have seen this as a glimmer of light on a horizon of anticipated future pain...

After a few decades of cautious experimentation with drugs for pain relief, the 1950s did more than revolutionise our tastes in music. Suddenly, Elvis and his contemporaries made sexually explicit and—more to the point—sexually *arousing* images socially acceptable. This, along with the introduction of the Pill in the early 1960s, was no doubt a key to the opening up of women's sexuality. Suddenly, women were not only able to control whether or not they had babies, they were even able to enjoy sex outside marriage. This put a whole new focus on their sexual activities. Instead of being something which was feared (with its inevitable consequences, in terms of pregnancies, injury and incontinence—not to mention death in some cases), it became something which could be enjoyed.

With increasing sexual enjoyment came a new awareness of the possibilities of childbirth. Some women, quite accidentally perhaps, started discovering that birth could actually be *pleasurable*. Considering labour from an emotional and hormonal point of view, it is quite easy to understand why this change in perception might have occurred. After all, fear triggers the production of adrenaline and this hormone makes the production of another hormone impossible—that hormone being oxytocin, which happens to be crucial to the progress of labour, since it causes contractions and makes possible not only cervical dilation, but also the birth of the baby. In a fearful environment, with the production of oxytocin stopped (because of the labouring woman's fear), it's hardly surprising that labours had often been hard and ineffective. If labours were not slowed down by fear, they would certainly have been slowed down by other interventions which had, by then, become commonplace: routine induction (meaning that many women were expected to have efficient labours when these had been triggered far too early) and, perhaps most importantly, the widespread immobilisation of labouring women, who were now expected to spend their labours in the least facilitative position possible, lying down on their backs, with their feet in stirrups. Not even gravity could come to their rescue and it's likely that—with artificial oxytocin increasingly being used to 'spur on' women's labours, the pain of childbirth was becoming insufferable.

But some women's new awareness and enjoyment of their sexuality was revealing a new perspective of labour and birth... In a supportive, happy, loving environment these women would have produced oxytocin, which has been called the 'hormone of love' (since it is produced in loving situations and during orgasm) and they would suddenly have started discovering new possibilities for birth. (Their labours would also have been far smoother and safer, which must have added to their relief.) The contemplations and writings of Grantley Dick-Read (who considered the role of fear in birth, after seeing a fearless woman experience no pain), Sheila Kitzinger (who encouraged women to see birth as a psycho-sexual experience), and Janet Balaskas (who got women back on their feet again, and moving around) helped this process along. Michel Odent's open-minded approach also helped to fuel a whole new movement because he observed that women who laboured in private, intimate environments had much smoother, safer labours. Suddenly, some people were not seeing drug-free birth as a sentence but as a solution. Perhaps a new type of labour was possible after all?

The advent of the epidural in the 1960s started up the debate all over again. Other forms of pain relief provided a middle ground for women who wanted to avoid the kind of high-level medicalisation which an epidural involves, or the possible risk. These options included and continue to include drugs such as 'gas and air' (which dentists 100 years ago were afraid to use on adults, because it sometimes caused death) and opiates such as pethidine and diamorphine... The fact that many research studies have shown increased incidence of many problems for the baby at birth or years later (e.g. in early adulthood) has not constituted much of a disincentive for women who are keen to avoid over-medicalisation but who—at the same time—want some form of relief from pain during labour and birth, which they still see as terrifying and unacceptable. And epidurals, the extremely medical alternative (which comes with its own increased risks for both mother and baby, according to research) have proved their worth as a substitute to general anaesthesia during caesarean sections.

Even caesareans have proved to be increasingly popular in the UK and around the world—with rates rising to 90% in some urban hospitals in Brazil and China. But, again, few women talk about the risks they involve, or the problems which too often occur postnatally. What's more, thanks to the increasing use of caesareans as an alternative to labour and thanks to negative birth mythology in the media, women again seem to be rediscovering their fear of days gone by. Not everyone has heard about or experienced the joys which some women report in ecstatic tones, and mentions of orgasmic births simply puzzle most people.

On the positive side, living in the UK in the 21st century, you have the luxury of choice. Irrespective of the relative safety or risks of the various options, the law allows you to choose to approach birth in whatever way you prefer. This means, if you're pregnant now, you have some important decisions to make. With her fascinating analysis of our cultural history, with her discussion of the role pain plays in our lives, with her description of our body's responses to pain, with her overview of historical developments and with her 30+ years of experience as a midwife, Verena Schmid should be able to guide you through this maze of choices... and help you reach a decision which is right for you.

Sylvie Donna

Introduction

The meaning of labour pain for modern women

The aim of this book is to give you a comprehensive overview of birth pain (including labour pain) and ways of dealing with it. This should make it possible for you to have a real choice, after you have weighed up your personal values and needs, and the pros and cons of each approach you read about.

We live in a time of rapid cultural change. Inevitably, there are difficulties with adjustment, a certain amount of inner disorientation and a kind of ambivalence between old and new ways. At this point in human history it is vital that information is made available and that we discuss and explore possibilities, so that we can come to a better understanding of birth. Every woman in the developed world now has real freedom to make choices about what is best for her, without being judged or treated with prejudice. Nevertheless, in order for this choice to be possible, you will need to use some new 'tools' and you will need to consider new interpretations of ancient birth paradigms.

In order for real choice to be possible, you will need to consider new interpretations of ancient birth paradigms

If we want to be freed from old approaches to care, we must first remember and understand our roots—the situations we started with and our point of departure. Only after this can we decide what to leave behind and what to bring to a new model of living, and only after remembering and understanding our roots can we interpret the meaning of our contemporary experience. What's more, a consideration of pain will involve considering profound existential topics. If, on the other hand, we were to ignore the issue of pain, this would mean *feeling* less and finding out less about ourselves.

Female authors such as Adrienne Rich (1976), Suzanne Arms (1975), Sheila Kitzinger (2008), Doris Haire (1972), Margaret Mead (2001), Ina May Gaskin (2008), as well as many others, have emphasised the importance of experiencing birth fully because birth is inextricably part of a woman's life and her sexuality and it influences the quality of both. Birth is therefore associated with female power, with her ability as a woman, with her strength, and also with her personal and social creativity.

Birth is inextricably part of a woman's life and her sexuality and it influences the quality of both

The definition of birth as a psychosexual event, the way in which hormones are produced as a result of pain and the growing sexual tension during labour all testify to the idea that motherhood and sexuality are intertwined. In my view, through the process of becoming a mother many old psychosexual traumas can be healed. Nevertheless, the rediscovery of birth as a transformative event has various, often demanding, implications... Compromises, adaptation, even disappointment, sacrifice in the form of suffering and personal as well as social limitations seem to be inevitable stages on the long path to motherhood.

Experiencing birth also means coming to grips with the art of survival, just as animals and plants need to understand survival. When the processes of reproduction and growth are only understood in terms of technology, with no concern for the primary relationship of the mother and Mother Earth, the art of giving birth will be in danger of being lost and it will already begin to die out... If it is lost, either wholly or partially, we will lose the very knowledge of life and survival. Considering birth in this way, we're not starting out with an idealised picture but with a reality with a complex history, which we want to understand more fully. Perhaps needless to say, an understanding of pain in relation to birth is an essential part of the understanding we need to develop, seeing birth within the context of its long and complex history across different cultures.

Verena Schmid

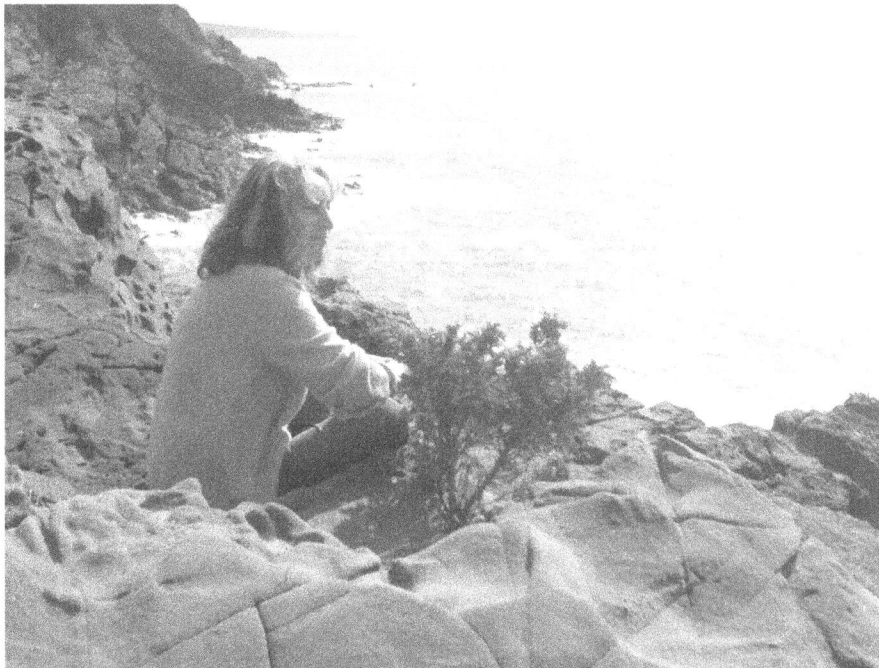

Verena relaxing by the sea...

CHAPTER 1:

Cultural influences on your experience of labour pain

Interpretations inspired by particular cultures

Pain is no doubt the most conspicuous aspect of childbirth, which—for hundreds and thousands of years up till the present day—has strangely attracted and fascinated some women, but inculcated fear, if not horror, in others. To the end of a woman's life women remember this aspect of childbirth which is an integral part of the experience of 'giving' birth.

In different cultures it is likely that pain is interpreted very differently and as a result its significance is conveyed very differently too. Pain associated with birth cannot be considered entirely separately because any kind of pain is deeply affected by the overriding philosophies of life underpinning any given society. How it is experienced is therefore dependent on the value negative sensations are generally assigned in a particular culture.

In many cultures pregnancy and birth are probably fear-inducing events which are considered 'unclean' quite simply because of their inherent power and capacity for endangering mother or child. At the same time, as Adrienne Rich noted in *Of Woman Born: Motherhood as Experience and Institution* (1976), pregnancy and birth are sometimes seen as processes which are susceptible to evil, as processes where evil originates or even as the embodiment of guilt. As a result, far-reaching significance is ascribed to these events which it is thought might, for example, endanger the annual harvest, evoke bad spirits or attract the evil eye. These processes are also sometimes seen as being the source of torment, or even—by contrast—a source of healing power, sexual power and much more.

The cultural anthropologist Margaret Mead (author of many books from the 1920s to the 1970s) noted that, depending on the culture, birth is seen as being either a painful and dangerous event, or an interesting, enriching experience (Mead, 2001). She said it is either seen as being individually determined or as something which arises as a result of a supernatural power. In some cultures the external expression of pain is tolerated, in others it is even encouraged, in yet others men mimic women's expression of pain and in some cultures it is not accepted at all. Here, again, in the field of childbirth we find that attitudes are a reflection of what is tolerated in a more generalised way, within society.

Attitudes to birth reflect society's values generally

Only a few anthropological studies have been conducted on childbirth simply because researchers, who are mainly men, are kept well away from the events of birth. They find out about difficult labours but know little about normal birth. Nevertheless, we can certainly assume that a society which lives in harmony with nature and which sees suffering as unavoidable and simply part of the normal, ongoing cycle of life will have more understanding and acceptance of labour pain and pain in general than a society which is not living in harmony with nature and its rhythms. Living in harmony with nature and being in tune with its rhythms, inspires all kinds of deep understandings. For example, a person with this world view understands that no state is static or eternal, whether it relates to happiness or suffering. With this outlook on life, it is understood that things are constantly changing and that one thing is always a prerequisite for the existence of something else. As a result, people who live in harmony with nature understand how to deal with constant changes and they accept them... and women giving birth in these cultures have this same understanding. Sometimes people even intentionally seek out pain in order to increase their own strength at times of growth, or when facing new tasks or responsibilities.

In women, each biological change is accompanied by some kind of physical or spiritual discomfort: the onset of menstruation (menarche), loss of virginity, childbirth, and sometimes even breastfeeding and the menopause. Men, by contrast, do not go through the same changes. Perhaps to compensate for their lack of natural transitional experiences, adult males in many societies have created numerous initiation rites to hail the arrival of puberty, marriage, fatherhood, war or a hunt – or some other important event. These rites involve men voluntarily subjecting themselves to discomfort and physical or psychological pain, or even inflicting injuries on themselves. Their reason for behaving in this way is that they know they become stronger and more powerful when they are able to survive physical and spiritual suffering.

In male activities such as war, conquests, adventures or expeditions, pain and even the struggle against death are accepted as a matter of course. A man prepares for an adventure and obtains any equipment, as necessary. He sets himself a challenge, with the aim of conquering something and emerging afterwards triumphant, stronger and wiser. His first thought is not about any pain he may suffer or about things going wrong; instead his full concentration is on whatever he is trying to achieve.

In some cultures, childbirth even seems to be seen as a kind of 'women's war'. Armed like soldiers, their eyes fixed on their goal, these women stride into labour. In societies which are more tuned in to nature it is assumed a woman will be expected to master the challenge of birth and it is also anticipated that she will emerge stronger and wiser from the whole experience. Birth is her personal business so she is likely to distance herself from society at this time in order to face her challenges alone, using her own strength. In other societies birth seems to be experienced as an ecstatic, transcendental event. When a woman surrenders to her own, instinctive abilities it then becomes a social, usually female, ritual, which facilitates personal growth and which, by constituting an ordeal in itself, triggers a complete transformation into a state of fulfilment.

People in industrialised societies live an intense lifestyle, geared to productivity. Within this lifestyle there is hardly room for anything irrational or for individual rhythms which are in tune with the cycles of nature. Time has a scientific value and it is goal-oriented. All physiological processes are supposed to take place in a linear fashion (with no 'ups' and 'downs') and they have only one thing as their goal: constant feelings of well-being, without any highs or lows. Within this view of life there is no room for pain and there is certainly no appreciation of it. The only kind of efforts recognised by many people are those which relate to financial achievement (Giddens, 1991; Giddens 1992).

The possibility of death shocks people and is shut out by promises implied by false safety measures. In this way any discomfort becomes linear too, i.e. it is not seen as part of a complex process, which is part of a cycle which involves challenges and rewards. Labour therefore loses its rhythm and then transmutes into chronic suffering because pain is interpreted as a sign of things getting progressively worse. Suffering and its ability to polarise things as part of the rhythm of life gets forgotten, alongside the possibility that pain can be *expressed* and lived through. When people deny the possibility of death and the reality of their own vitality, they also lose the experience of life's depths. In my view in our society a technological, linear model of birth, without any rhythm or contrasts, characterised by chronic discomfort or trauma, takes precedence.

However... will a different kind of society—a society like ours, in which women are denied the experience of birth pain, breastfeeding, traumatic change and emotional pain—end up producing weaker women? And in a society where men no longer accept or even seek out real challenges aren't men also weaker? In our lives today isn't there a distinct lack of peak experiences?

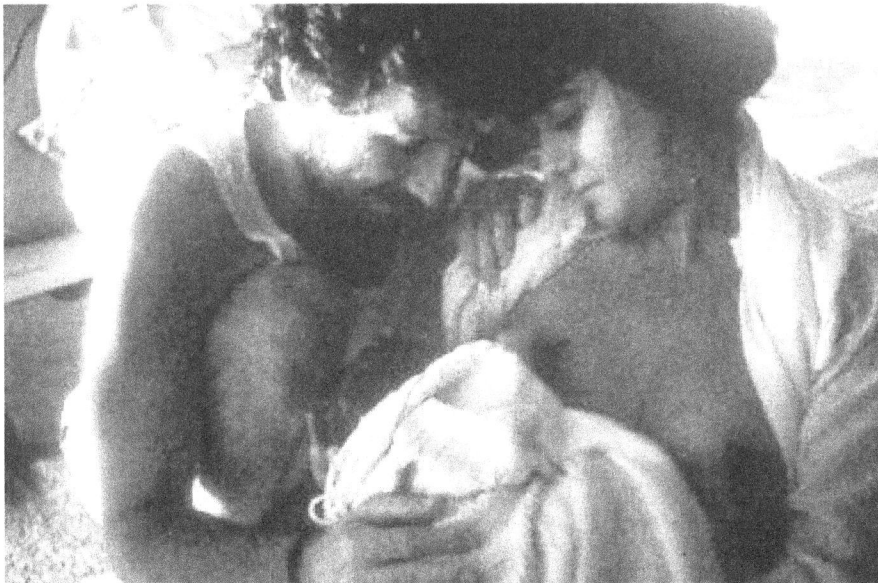

A couple sharing the challenging but also fulfilling experience of birth

Pain seen as punishment and eternal damnation

In Western societies, the idea of torment through biblical damnation seems to be indelibly etched on people's minds. This idea is often mentioned when pain relief is justified and it seems to embody the idea within society that motherhood should also be a kind of 'social sacrifice'. It seems to me that women are forced to decide between motherhood and a career, between becoming 'frumpy' mums and adults who express their creativity. They have to choose whether they are going to live as a hemmed-in mother or as a free agent, whether they are going to be a mother or a lover, a saint or a whore... and so it goes on.

Of course, modern women refuse to accept the notion of damnation. It's no longer seen as acceptable to see childbirth as punishment for a woman's sins, particularly sexual ones. Modern women try to distance themselves from the traditional model of passive suffering, which they see as outdated, in whatever way they can. And women who are no longer prepared to passively accept traditional ideas feel the need to demand liberation—and this often expresses itself in the form of requests for 'painfree birth', which is supposedly achieved with the help of an epidural.

The epidural 'solution' nevertheless means that a woman must behave passively during a potentially creative event; it means that motherhood becomes divorced from sexuality because all sensual aspects of birth, including the strong sexual tension of the birth act, get shut out along with the pain. Ideas based on the biblical idea of suffering in childbirth therefore remain unchanged... Perhaps it will help us to eradicate our preconceptions about birth if we consider an alternative interpretation of the biblical story of Eve, which will allow us to re-evaluate the experience of childbirth.

In this different interpretation of the creation, I would like to translate the traditional story into symbolic language. We could see Eden as an embodiment of the spiritual, natural world, which is ruled by unity, harmony and peace. We could see Eden as being the place of our origin, the mother's womb. Nevertheless, this place contains no possibility of experiencing duality (good and evil) or of developing consciousness. The serpent represents intuition, which offers Eve (through the apple) both knowledge and consciousness. Eve offers this knowledge to Adam, the male, and he accepts. In fact, men need women or the female part of themselves in order to reach consciousness. Banishment from Eden represents the transition to the physical world and the entrance into the world of contrasts, i.e. it represents birth. During this process the spiritual world becomes hidden, and the birth itself marks the beginning of the experience of human life, emerging consciousness and development through contrasts and recurring rhythms. In this view, men achieve self-actualisation mainly by working, doing things in the physical world and by providing for loved ones in material terms, or in other words, through social challenges and achievement. With women, during their fertile years, birth could be seen as a kind of initiation, and as a means to personal change or even transformation.

Rhythmic pain is a means towards deeper contrasts, deeper understanding, deeper emotions, consciousness, transcendence, ecstasy and development.

Of course these male and female contrasts—which I shall refer to as 'polarities'—occur in both men and women's lives. Nevertheless, women have more ways of reaching transcendental states, because they don't only experience their sexuality (as men do), but they may also experience birth and breastfeeding.

Photo © Sandro Pintus

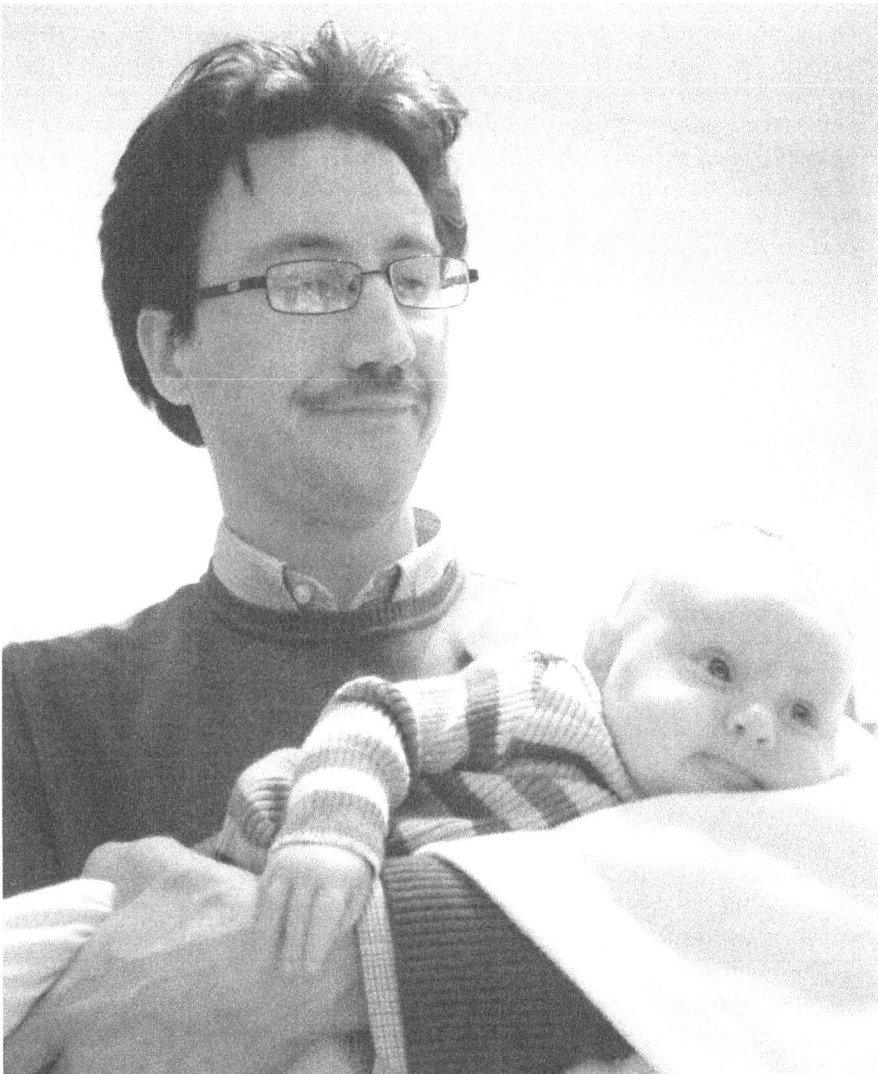

It's always useful to consider these issues with the baby in mind too

Pain seen as a gift for both you and your child

Using this more modern interpretation of the story in Genesis in the Bible, we can see the pain of childbirth not as a form of damnation, but as a *gift,* a privilege, or an opportunity. This is also how the indigenous people of North America—for example, the Cherokees—view pain in birth. They say that pain represents a gift for women because each uterine contraction helps to create the gift of new life and brings women nearer to their greatest wish, which is to have a child. Contractions are also a 'gift' for the baby because they teach him or her the rhythms of life and prepare him or her for life in this world.

In some societies the higher state of consciousness which arises during childbirth can even become transformed into euphoria. Jeannine Parvati Baker said that when a woman is experienced in doing spiritual exercises, which involve giving up the ego and reaching higher states of consciousness as well as oneness with the universe, she can give birth overcoming the pain. Parvati Baker explains that this is because she will let herself be led by contractions and not resist them. This will in turn mean she can move towards the birth of her child with no pain and that she can experience the actual event in a state of ecstasy (Parvati Baker, 1987).

Clearly, in some cultures, rituals and ceremonies before and during birth help to open the way for the child and they therefore support the process of childbirth. Singing, flute-playing and certain rhythmical instruments are used in some cultures and these promote a hypnotic state of mind. Even poetry reading and the stimulation of increased awareness through the use of aromas, images and sounds are used in some places to promote opening because these all stimulate the right side of the brain, which governs birth as well as our creativity.

The false promise of a painfree birth

When considering spontaneous birth and also how childbirth is organised in a society, we have to take into account the lifestyle a woman and her family enjoys, because this affects the way she gives birth. In addition we need to understand that a society's general values are reflected in the way in which births are planned. People experiencing a monotonous lifestyle, without ups and downs, in a technologically oriented society which is disconnected from female cyclical changes, will choose a birth which is linear, in terms of industrial and technological measurements. People who feel more connected to nature will seek out a physiological birth, following a cyclic rhythm through labour and they will try to 'go with the flow'. Furthermore, women who strive for excellence, who accept life's cyclical processes, will choose to give birth as consciously as possible.

A linear way of living always attempts to shut out negative feelings, and people who live this way are always surprised when suddenly one of life's rhythms makes itself felt. When a woman living a life which has been planned in a linear fashion faces these very real experiences, she is totally unprepared. She feels divided between her inner, instinctive model of birth and that which society imposes as normal. As a result, a conflict emerges between two profound needs: the need to follow one's instincts, and the need to belong to a group. Since, in this case, biological needs are in conflict with cultural needs the woman feels frustrated and inadequate in terms of her existence as a woman and mother. She is confused, so she seeks help from experts.

Let us now take the example of a technological birth, which takes place with an epidural sited. The promise of a painfree birth cannot be kept in reality. This is not only because epidurals are not available to all women, it's also because they can only be administered when the active phase of labour has begun. This means that women simply have to come to grips with the idea of pain. But they aren't prepared for this and they struggle against pain, so suffer all the more keenly. What's more, postnatally they don't experience intense satisfaction from endorphins, which they would if they were to have a physiological birth. The lack of endorphins from birth results in more painful sensations after the birth. And the lack of a feeling of satisfaction reduces or prevents any wish to repeat the experience and have other children.

In reality, labour cannot be avoided on the journey into motherhood. When attempts are made to 'simplify' the birth process and its dynamics by suppressing pain and therefore also hormonal production, these processes have to be faced later on without facilitative hormones, so recovery, convalescence and the relationship with the baby are much more difficult.

Brigitte Jordan surveyed how birth takes place in four different cultures (Jordan, 1992). She showed that women who suffer most during childbirth are those who have been falsely promised they can have a so-called 'painfree' birth with the help of an epidural. These women are unprepared for the early pain of labour and unmotivated to face it so it is perceived as being worse than later pain in labour experienced by other women. This is partly because the compensatory mechanisms (of endorphin production) only properly kick in during the active stage of labour. By contrast, women who suffer the least are the ones who are motivated and prepared for pain and feel ready to put up with it. This is particularly the case when their social environment also shares this attitude and accepts pain. In fact, pain becomes considerably worse when women try and suppress it. It becomes manageable when it is accepted without protest.

It seems to me that labour often becomes pathological when birth attendants, who are frequently seen as a guarantee of safety, take complete control of birth. Risks arise as a result of medical intervention—as we shall see, when we consider the side-effects of drug-based forms of pain relief—and caregivers' interventions create problems which may continue long after the birth has taken place. These problems may include loss of sensitivity, permanent injuries to the central nervous system, and backache. With the technological management of birth, risks and problems also increase, instead of being reduced, as is promised, and this, along with caregivers' tendency to intervene tends to make labouring and birthing women very passive. In reality, surprisingly perhaps, it seems that women therefore suffer more in societies which are focused on wellbeing.

In our society, where birth is perhaps the last remaining conscious transition in life, it is sometimes helpful for us to use positive rituals, even during pregnancy. These can strengthen us, while we are pregnant, and also prepare us for an event which is far from the everyday experience of life, which is perhaps nevertheless awaited deep within every woman. After all, without any doubt, the experience of childbirth can constitute a real high or low point in a woman's life. The experience has enormous significance for a woman's future life because it makes a deep impression on her, which cannot be avoided. If we also consider how this event is charged with centuries of memory and— because of the decreasing birth rate in developed countries— that it can be experienced less and less often, we will realise that it is perhaps worthwhile going beyond what is generally known and to think about a few issues relating to birth, instead of simply letting things passively take their course.

We need to tap into our deep-seated motivation, our ability to go with the flow of sensations, as well as into our ability to be aware of the child inside us, because this can be a great help to us. Childbirth is no longer something most women can do as a matter of course... It is something that we must rediscover. What we relearn as a result is useful not only for birth, but also for our lives afterwards with children, who are still very much in tune with nature in the early days of their lives.

Fear of pain, fear as a vehicle of oppression

Fear definitely exists! It is a physiological reaction to danger. It increases alertness and a person's ability to react quickly and constitutes an emotional response to tension. In labour it exists partly because of the unknown aspects of birth, partly because of reports of negative experiences heard from other women, and partly because of social conditioning. We may experience various fears, for example we may be afraid of losing self-control, we may be afraid of the strength of our own feelings, we may be afraid of exposing ourselves, of being inadequate or weak, we may be afraid that we ourselves will die, or that our baby will be damaged or stillborn, or we may simply be afraid of 'losing' ourselves somehow.

Some fears are ontogenetic, i.e. they are specific to certain people or cultures, while other fears are phylogenetic, i.e. they are primal fears which are similar in all women and relate to the act of giving birth itself (Martin and Murray, 2008). Whatever type it is, fear is certainly a *physiological* reaction to danger. It increases alertness and a person's ability to react quickly and constitutes an emotional response to tension, which arises as a result of labour pain.

There seem to be various ways of reacting to fear... If it is suppressed, it transmutes into anxiety or physical illness. If it is passively endured, it leads to affliction. If it is projected, it has an impact on other people (i.e. it 'contaminates' them), while the person him- or herself feels protected from its full internal effect. If, on the other hand, a fear is faced head on and acknowledged, it can be dissolved.

Caregivers are also susceptible to the dynamics of birth

Even people who attend pregnant and labouring women are susceptible to the same dynamics. They can distance themselves from women's fears and their own using techniques to control them. They can let themselves be contaminated by women's fears, which I would suggest often results in them misusing their own power in order to dominate women (and their own fear). Alternatively, they can face fears alongside pregnant or labouring women and use appropriate ways of helping them dissolve them.

Simone Weil described the difference between suffering and despondency (Rich, 1996). She said that suffering which is characterised by pain leads to a maturation process and recognition. She then contrasted this with pain which is avoided, saying that this kind leads to affliction, the condition of oppressed people such as the inmates of a concentration camp, who were forced to carry loads to and fro for no reason whatsoever. She sees affliction as being on the same level as impotence, indecision, disintegration and inactivity. She said pain is not something to seek out, but when it's inevitable it can be transformed into 'something useful' which allows us to go beyond our previous limitations, and get to know the possibilities in our lives much better... It therefore seems to me that people can avoid depression by actively confronting fear and pain.

In certain cultures, women's fear has been used and promoted in order to establish the supremacy of powerful people over women, e.g. by miracle workers, doctors and priests. By keeping women caught up in their own fear and reducing their ability to respond effectively to this emotion, it is possible to manipulate and control women for purposes which might be scientific, social, religious or personal.

Acceptance of pain, acceptance of means to freedom

If we actively accept pain in labour, we will inevitably need to work and seek out new ways of being in order to promote a process of learning. This means we will need to be alert to possibilities and that we will need to explore and use different approaches to pain management. However, we need to be aware that it only makes sense to do this in the context of physiological birth in certain conditions, specifically when you have the freedom to move and express yourself. Otherwise, you would be accepting unproductive pain, and there would be no point in this. When you are labouring in the right conditions, the acceptance of pain may take place spontaneously—if you yourself have already experienced a gentle birth or if your mother was left with a positive impression of the whole experience.

In 1975, in the book *Immaculate Deception* (Houghton Mifflin, 1975), Suzanne Arms wrote that after centuries of fear, expectation of pain and obedience to male control systems, women cannot suddenly launch into childbirth as a completely new woman (with a new outlook) after only a couple of hours of antenatal preparation or a pep talk about feminism (Arms, 1975).

When we give birth, we can only take along with us to the experience what we are as women already. This is bound to be a mixture of the old and the new. As well as accepting labour pain as a way of having a conscious experience, we also need to behave *as if we are a leading lady* in a play... In other words, we need to be completely free in terms of how we express ourselves. Our needs are encapsulated in the term 'active birth', which was originally coined by Janet Balaskas (founder of the Active Birth Centre in London) (Balaskas, 1994). An active birth means that you are in contact with your body, that you can freely express yourself and be at the centre of the situation, alongside your partner and baby. Working towards an acceptance of pain strengthens this view of birth, which is suppressed in most women today.

A Catch-22 situation

Nowadays, various methods for relieving pain are suggested to women having normal births and a birth involving analgesia or anaesthesia is presented as being much better than a birth involving pain. Originally, though, pain relief was only recommended during difficult labours. The tendency nowadays to encourage women to see drug-based pain relief as the best way forward is widespread in the UK, the USA, Germany and France and it's becoming increasing common in Italy, where I live and work. Pain relief is less in demand in Holland, which has retained a relatively 'natural' birth culture, compared to other European countries. Since women's groups in Italy have called for the 'right' to have an epidural it has become an established political goal there to increase the epidural rate nationwide to at least 30%. However, medical approaches to pain relief communicate to us that our body is a machine, which functions better with technological support. This is a misleading message.

The widespread acceptance of pain killers is based on the view that the body and mind are separate. This leads to a ritual which emphasises women's disconnection from reproductive processes. And sensitivity towards one's own body, harmony between physical processes and emotional experience, between mother and child, the rhythmical flow of pain and the experience of transformation are no longer seen as valuable and worth striving for. This is because they would remind people of their dependence on nature, their vulnerability and their helplessness in the face of bodily functions. Medical technology aims to control nature and make it her servant so that women can hide their weakness. This is why medical technology tries to shut out pain... Nevertheless, in the process of doing that we are left feeling unaware of our strength and that strength is then lost.

Medical technology tries to shut out pain because its purpose is to try and control nature and hide weakness

In many cases the alternative to an epidural is still an alienated birth with acutely unnatural pain. This is because immobility, unnatural postures and medical interventions make us afraid, lonely and make us feel abandoned, alone, trapped, helpless, and robbed of our own personality. Things get even worse if there is inadequate help and support and if we feel that we are being penalised or treated in an inhumane way. (So-called 'family-friendly' or 'mother-friendly' hospitals are fortunately more readily available now, but there are still far too few of them.) The pain which occurs in these unfavourable conditions is certainly impossible to justify. In these conditions the high demand for pain killers is more than understandable and legitimate, but, in fact, in these circumstances, we are not really exercising any freedom of choice. We're simply in a Catch-22 situation. After all, we need the pain relief because of the situation we're in. In order to be able to cope with normal birth pain, it is necessary to have a supportive environment.

Without a supportive environment, drugs are needed

Adrienne Rich wrote that modern forms of pain relief are creating a new type of prison for women: a prison of unconscious experience, clouded perception, forgetfulness and total passivity. She went on to say that running away from physical or spiritual pain sets off a dangerous mechanism, which involves not only no longer being in contact with painful sensations, but also no longer being in touch with oneself (Rich, 1976). I would add, that even medicalised hospital birth lying down, attached to a monitor, without one-to-one support represents being in a kind of prison. We need a new way of coping with birth and normal labour pain, so that we can leave this prison which our modern culture has created.

In many places—in the USA, Latin America and Italy—there isn't really any freedom of choice for women since natural approaches to dealing with pain and professional support during labour and birth are not generally offered. In these places, the epidural represents the medical approach to birth. To health care professionals, it may be an easy option because women don't need to be supported, or at least that may be what many professionals think. Since there are few midwives in hospitals or only nurses, traditional or independent woman-centred midwives only attend births outside the hospital environment.

At first glance, the situation does at least seem better in Britain because here there are many committed midwives, who make an enormous effort to provide a service which is 'friendly' to women, babies and families. But even these midwives experience their limitations all too often as a result of institutional problems, conflicts with colleagues and hierarchies, which make it impossible to change certain things, which 'have always been done like that'. It's possible that financial factors may also be significant in preventing positive change from taking place.

In any case, there are very few studies which compare epidurals with non-drug-based methods of pain relief so it is cultural influences which determine the choices we make or the care we are given and the way in which we experience labour pain, not data from scientific studies. Having said that, while many cultures worldwide are now tending to encourage a drug-based approach to pain relief, some midwives and women are opting for methods of pain relief which do not involve drugs. This makes sense because early data from research certainly does indicate potential problems with drug-based forms of pain relief. The move 'back' to drug-free, natural approaches also makes sense, given the physiological causes of pain and its probable functions during labour and birth—as we shall see in the next chapter.

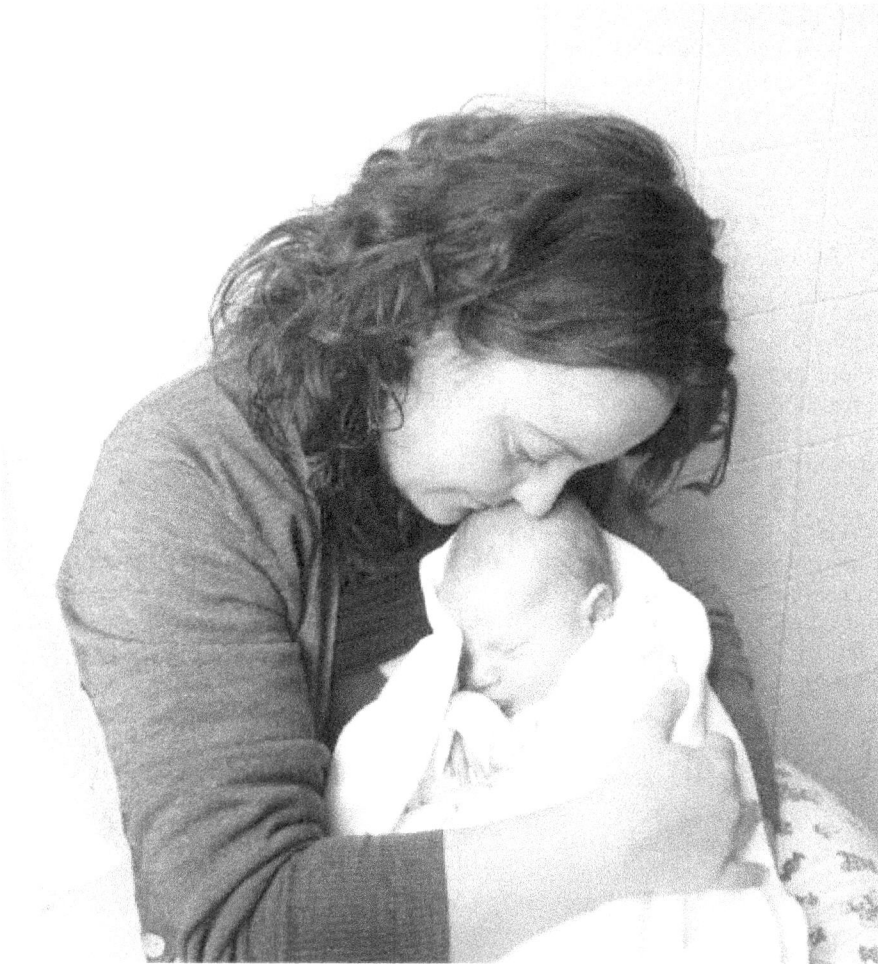

A new mother with her newborn, both of them travelling through the physiological processes of pregnancy, birthing and breastfeeding, without artificial support

CHAPTER 2:

Physiological principles and the functions of labour pain

The function of pain in physiological labour

All natural, physiological processes in our bodies are painfree. If one of these processes—for example, our breathing or digestion—becomes painful, any pain we experience functions as a warning signal. The founders of psychoprophylaxis (the Russian form of pain control in labour) have therefore long debated whether labour pain should be regarded as natural (physiological), or if it should be seen as a sign of pathology. Chertok and Langen (1968), suggested that the experience of pain during labour is an expression of female neurosis and a figment of their imagination. They therefore argued that some 80% of women should have psychotherapy before giving birth.

When studying painfree spontaneous births Agnetti (1992) found that between 7% and 14% of women in Western countries give birth without experiencing any pain. This percentage is similar to the number of people who would easily fall into a deep state of hypnosis during hypnotherapy. Research has yet to be conducted to establish whether there is a link between these two sets of results. However, it would be easy to hypothesise that there is indeed a connection because birth involves going into an altered state of consciousness or at least involves the ability to easily let oneself go. Women who can easily move into a trance-like state could perhaps have a different or significantly reduced perception of pain. After all, Jeannine Parvati Baker wrote that giving birth consciously is the ultimate spiritual practice, requiring purity in strength, flexibility, health, concentration, surrender and faith (Parvati Baker, 2001).

For the vast majority of women birth is nevertheless painful. Pain could well be seen to have an evolutionary function: during labour pain forces the woman to be very aware of the event and it therefore serves to protect both mother and child. This idea becomes even more convincing when we see birth as being a paradoxical physiological process, when we see childbirth as being an attack on our integrity. In other words, in order to give life to another human being we have to do something which goes against the best interests of our body. We must endure a baby's attack on our very innards, which naturally goes against our instinct for self-preservation. Such an 'attack' on our personal integrity puts our body into a state of alarm. Pain then signals to our body that we are in danger and forces it to react. In a certain way childbirth therefore represents a battle between self-preservation and self-sacrifice. The unselfishness of the act of giving birth is nevertheless balanced out (in the case of a drug-free physiological birth, which involves no augmentation) by an enormous sense of satisfaction postnatally, which makes us want to repeat the experience—to give birth again and have more children.

The nature of labour pain

One of the most noticeable features of labour pain is its rhythmic nature. The rhythm consists of pain followed by breaks, contraction and release, discomfort and well-being, through acceleration followed by a slowing down. This rhythm is dynamic and may change under the influence of various individual factors. Its tempo is dependent on our own personality and experiences and the baby being born, so cannot be defined in a general way.

Labour pain is therefore intermittent pain with an individual dynamic, which varies according to our needs and those of our baby. In its rhythmical nature lies one of the greatest mysteries of physiological birth and physiological pain management. This is what makes it intrinsically different from other types of pain. The changing rhythms over the course of a particular labour allow both mother and child to gradually adapt to what is happening. If this very specific rhythm is not respected and labour is augmented this will mean increased stress for us, as well as for the baby.

Pain triggers

Pain emanates from two places (Bonica, 1977; Melzack, 1973; Melzack and Wall, 1989). On the one hand it comes from the physical body, from the part where the attack on our integrity is taking place, i.e. on the periphery of the pelvis. On the other hand, pain comes from the brain, specifically from the area responsible for our feelings, sensations, instincts and the subconscious... from the place where our experience of life is stored. Peripheral areas stimulate central pain receptors and both the peripheral stimuli and the response from the brain work together to produce an individual person's experience of pain.

THE SENSITIVE PERIPHERAL (OR 'PHYSICAL') TRIGGERS

The uterus and the cervix accommodate many sensitive nerve endings, which—in conjunction with the sympathetic nerves—can be traced back to the spinal cord. This utero-cervical and pelvic nerve plexus (neural network) is connected to the hypogastric nerves, which go round the broad ligaments of the uterus and through nerve pathways to the outer labia, all of these being part of the front of the pelvis and the straight pelvic muscles. This network follows the iliac crest and then joins the superior hypogastric plexus (i.e. the presacral nerve), ending in the pathways of the sympathetic nervous system in the lumbar region, under the thorax. From there, the pathways lead out from spinal nerves, thoracic nerves 11 (Th 11) and 12 (Th 12) and from there on even further to thoracic nerves 10 and lumbar nerve 1 (L 1).

The skin nerve endings over the 11th thoracic nerves (Th 11) stimulate the skin lying over the area of the 3rd and 4th lumbar vertebrae, extending from the spinal cord. Nerve endings in the 12th thoracic nerves innervate the skin over the 5th vetebra and the first sacral vertebra. The branching off of the hypogastric nerve innervates the skin at the front of the body, underneath the lower abdomen.

Therefore, the pain we feel as a result of uterine contractions is felt on the surface of the skin in the same way as any other kind of internal pain (i.e. visceral pain), which is innervated by the same area of the spine. After all, although there are numerous local receptors in muscle tissue in the lower segment of the uterus and the cervix, these only register pain in the case of injury or overstretching. By contrast, there are very few receptors in the fundus. As a result, we mainly feel labour pain in the lower part of the abdomen, on the side of the iliac crest and at the back, in the area of the sacrum. The pelvis, vagina and coccyx are all innervated by the pudendal and coccygeal nerves. These branch off into the pelvic nerves, which also serve the bladder, rectum and vagina. The pudendal nerve runs through the ischiorectal fossa up to the 2nd, 3rd and 4th sacral vertebrae (within the spinal cord).

Physical factors influencing labour pain

Here we are talking about internal pain, which occurs as a result of overstretching, tears and also ischemia in the uterine muscles (i.e. an insufficiency of blood supply in this localised area). (Note, though, that the latter—ischemia—does not occur in undrugged, physiological labours, where the contractions are rhythmic and where spaces between contractions involve complete relaxation.) In particular, labour pain results from the following physical causes:

- Overstretching of the cervix and tiny tears in this area. There is a close connection between the intensity of pain and the opening of the cervix, especially when the cervix is very rigid.
- Strain in the lower uterine segment.
- Pulled ligaments.
- Pressure on nerve endings in the lumbosacral plexus (in the area of the lumbar vertebrae and the sacrum).
- Pressure on the pelvic joints.
- Opening, tearing and stretching of the pelvic ligaments and the vulva. The intensity of pain is directly proportional to the degree of tension or relaxation in this sensitive area. The experience of pain during the second stage of labour varies enormously from one woman to another—from strong pain to a simple feeling of exertion.
- Ischemia of the uterine muscles occurs as a result of metabolic over-oxygenation (acidosis) when contractions are either too frequent or too long, i.e. when contractions are unnatural. Normal uterine contractions are not painful in the upper part of the uterus.

THE CENTRAL (OR 'PSYCHOLOGICAL') TRIGGERS

Research has shown that the experience of pain is not simply the result of the perception of a peripheral trigger, followed by a reaction when this message is conveyed along a pain pathway to a pain centre in the brain (Melzack, 1989).

In fact, the reasons why pain is experienced seem to be much more complex. Experiencing acute pain appears to be influenced by both physiological and psychological factors. The experience seems to involve most of the nervous system concerned with sensory perception, emotions, instincts, cognitive and motor processes, as well as psychodynamic mechanisms. Furthermore, central factors influencing the perception of pain can have the effect of either minimising or amplifying messages received from peripheral triggers.

Psychological factors influencing labour pain

- **Negative conditioning through unfavourable cultural circumstances** This kind of conditioning can include contempt for the procreative process of birth, poor self-esteem, early traumatic experiences in life. It can even simply be the result of hearing horror stories about birth, or of a negative perception of our own social role as a woman.
- **Environmental conditioning** This is to do with the way in which pain is viewed in our culture (either being valued, or being seen as something to avoid), the way in which birth and womanhood are experienced socially, the tendency (or not) for women to be compliant and passive, the attention paid to pain and the way in which people in a society usually proceed when pain occurs.
- **Personal life experience** This involves all painful personal experiences, including experiences of loss, the way in which you relate to yourself, your fears, emotional baggage left as a result of unresolved problems, your sexuality, your view of changes in life, your emotional maturity, your difficulties facing pain generally, or it can be the consequence of your painful experience of your own birth (as a baby), for example.

Psychological factors influence the way pain is felt

Pain pathways

Various nerve receptors are activated by the smallest possible impulse (beyond a threshold level), according to the laws of each type of receptor. Responses from the nerve receptors vary with increasingly descending inhibitive mechanisms. Stimuli pass along the sensitive fibres in the sympathetic nervous system, over visceral nerves in the parasympathetic nervous system and somatic nerves in the central nervous system to the spine (the posterior horns). The grey matter of the posterior horns prepares peripheral information obtained and transmits it to the brain.

The gelatinous substance of the posterior horns in the spine provides a kind of gateway to painful stimuli, which can open or close, either holding back stimuli or facilitating their transmission. What happens depends on the impulses, which the brain sends after receiving information by way of fast-transmission fibres (which are activators of central control).

THE GATE CONTROL THEORY OF PAIN

Melzack and Wall (1989) developed the theory of gate control, which they propose takes place in the grey matter (nerve cells) of the posterior horns of the spinal cord. These researchers claim that various complex control mechanisms take place at this place, under the influence of rising and falling impulses, and that information is exchanged and codes modified. The grey matter at the posterior horn, which is shaped like a butterfly, is surrounded by white matter and the researchers suggest that this is where the rising and falling and interactive pathways carry out their tasks.

The posterior horns are comprised of six different layers. In the first and second layers there is gelatinous substance of Rolando. This is a dense network of interwoven short fibres which receive messages from fibres of every kind coming from all over your body (even from other layers of the posterior horns). Melzack and Wall claim the network's important function is to modulate information. This involves a highly specialised, self-contained system of cells, which influences the activity of the nerve cells carrying stimuli to your brain.

The cells in the first and second layer receive stimuli from the A-delta fibres and C-fibres. The A-delta fibres are thick, pithy nerve fibres which speedily convey messages to your spinal cord and brain. They are also linked to high-threshold receptors so that vivid, well-localised acute pain can be identified. The C-fibres are thin, long, marrow-free extensions to your spine, which transmit stimuli over the reticular system to your thalamus, effectively sending messages about dull, bad, localised, or long-lasting pain, which prompts a slow reaction. They are linked to nocireceptors with free nerve endings. The C-fibres incorporate a high number of receptors for opiates, which are naturally produced in your body when you labour without any drugs in your system.

An intensively noxious (i.e. harmful) stimulus activates the A-delta fibres, involving a high number of C-fibres too, and increases the intensity of stimulation of all receptor fibres. Today it is assumed that you only perceive pain as occurring when the entire stimulation of stimulated nerve fibres has exceeded a certain critical level.

To summarise, the gate control theory of pain is based on several key ideas. The transmission of nerve stimuli from the periphery of your body to your spine is influenced by a control mechanism which is situated in the posterior horns. This spinal control mechanism is activated by the activity of the thick and thin fibres. The activity of the thick fibres prevents further transmission (since the entrance is closed off), while the activity of the thin fibres facilitates it (since the gateway is wide open). The spinal control mechanism is influenced by decreasing nerve impulses which come from your brain and which can either facilitate or block stimuli (by either opening or closing the gateway). A special system of fibres with a wide diameter and fast transmission speed (A-delta fibres) activates selective processes in your brain. As a result, the working of the gate control system is influenced by inhibiting pathways. (This involves the activation of central control.) As soon as conveyor cells in your spine exceed a critical level of stimulation, your central activation system is activated. This system involves each area of nerves and leads to the complex and characteristic behaviour model of pain.

According to this theory, thin fibres fulfil an important function in transmitting messages about pain to your brain. As soon as a harmful stimulus reaches a large number of thin fibres, these convey the stimulus and create conditions to bundle together these increasing stimuli. This leads to an intense discharge of conveyor cells in your spine, which can exceed the critical threshold level. Beyond this, the impulses in thin fibres are receptive to an alteration in activity of the whole nervous system. Thick fibres, by contrast, inhibit the transmission of stimuli to your brain. In this way the control mechanism in your spine is regulated by the antagonistic effect of the thick fibres with a small diameter, as well as by the limiting or stimulating effect of the inhibiting nerve fibres. Modulation of pain therefore takes place *before* it is perceived! Because of the effect of the central mechanism a painful stimulus can be strengthened, weakened or neutralised.

According to Melzack and Wall (1989) the nerve pathways which run along the spinal cord to the brain differentiate themselves by being either fast-output or slow-output. There are also pathways which inhibit and control pain.

THE FAST-OUTPUT PATHWAYS

The lemniscal system bundles together the fibres which emerge from the posterior horns of your spinal cord and transmits stimuli to your thalamus and to your parietal cortex (cerebral cortex). This system is made up of thick fibres and activates central control. Because the transmission speed of this lemniscal system is very high your brain can selectively perceive, evaluate, localise and modulate sensitive information before the various action systems (i.e. motor or vegetative systems) are activated. (The latter are explained on page 26.)

The spinothalamic tract comes to the fore in the anterior strangury system. It carries impulses to your thalamus and parietal cortex, your reticular system, your intrathalamic nuclei and your limbic system. In addition, it creates a connection with your hypothalamus, your pituitary gland and your vegetative nuclei. (As explained earlier, this is the traditional pain pathway.)

THE SLOW-OUTPUT PATHWAYS

The slow-output pathways are a network of short fibres bound together, running up your spinal cord and ending in your reticular system. Increasing stimuli are already influenced and modulated by the inhibiting control system. In terms of intensity these slow-output pathways are not necessarily in step with the intensity of the peripheral stimuli. In the same way as pain can already be experienced either before a stimulus has occurred, or even in the absence of any stimulus from the periphery of your body (merely because of fear or the expectation of pain), sensations may also *not* be perceived as pain, even when strong peripheral stimuli are in evidence.

DESCENDING PATHWAYS WHICH INHIBIT PAIN

These run through the pyramidals and extrapyramidal motor pathways, which are linked to your sympathetic and parasympathetic nervous system and end in the front lateral part of your spinal cord.

Descending inhibitive control systems

Your reticular system (formation reticularis) becomes involved with and analyses increasing stimuli from the periphery of your body and central stimuli from your cerebral cortex and limbic system. It connects these stimuli to your knowledge of life (gained from your experience), in order to then send inhibiting impulses to your posterior horns. There, the rising pain stimulus is first modified, before it is transmitted to various other regions of your brain, and a specific response follows. (This is the system which controls the level of intensity.)

Centrally stimulating conditions such as, for example, fear, arousal or other feelings, can therefore either open up or close off the relevant afferents in your body, using the barriers in your posterior horns. It can be assumed that your inhibiting control system uses serotonin as a neurotransmitter.

Muscular rigidity and lack of movement, for example, stimulate your reticular system pathologically and throw your cerebrum into a state of alarm. As a result, the sensitivity of all central structures relating to afferent stimuli is increased and in this way extreme reactions are provoked. This is why the expectation of pain increases the experience of pain. On the other hand, physiological movement of your muscles, involving relaxed muscle tone, stimulates your brain structures in a positive way, activates the inhibiting mechanisms (relating to sensory stimuli) and supports the production of endorphins and encephalins. This constitutes the natural pain relief, which is produced by your body.

Central mechanisms of pain

The *reticular system* (formation reticularis) extends the length of your spinal cord (medulla oblongata) right up to your interbrain, with some extension to your neocortex, and consists of a network of fibres, interwoven with clusters of cells. It is connected to your entire cranial nervous system, the amplifying and inhibiting pathways and in this way it stretches into all areas of your brain. This is where all kinds of information come together.

The reticular system modulates the strength of the stimuli and is therefore the actual intensity control system. Depending on the overall intensity of the stimulus, it either activates those areas of your brain which create pleasant feelings and the tendency to accept what is happening or—when stimuli exceed a certain critical threshold—it stimulates those areas of your brain which are responsible for unpleasant feelings and the tendency to refuse to go on. Your reticular system then sends inhibiting or amplifying impulses to all levels of the afferent pathways.

Your reticular system therefore puts your brain into a state of alertness and alarm, or into a state of depression and inhibition. It stimulates your pituitary gland and the production of adrenocorticotropic hormone (ACTH) and endorphins (which control all your sensory systems), it plays a fundamental role in integrating pain and behaviour and it is also important in the central controlling of increasing (afferent) information.

It is possible to see the increasing and decreasing pathways at the intersection of the peripheral stimuli and the centre of your brain as two currents in the sea, which meet up. At the point where both currents flow into each other there is swirling eddy of waves of different strengths, which are also affected by the strength of the currents. Then—after the two currents have come together and become mixed up—they both flow together in a rapid and powerful eddy of movement.

The limbic system is an archaic part of your brain and it is the seat of unconscious feelings and emotions, i.e. the total of human feelings and mental experience. It comprises the cingulate gyrus, the hippocampus, the amygdaloid body (the amygdala), the septum and the tegmental nuclei and carries impulses over to your thalamus and your hypothalamus. A few of its areas communicate directly with your frontal cortex. The stimulation of this limbic system can provoke a 'drawing-back' reaction or an attempt to run away, in order to evade stimulation. It attributes to stimuli either a pleasant, affective or unpleasant, traumatic meaning. The changing effect of your limbic and reticular systems is of special significance for the processing of pain. The level of intensity in your limbic system (which depends on suppressed, unconscious feelings and unresolved problems) determines reactions to pain.

The thalamus is positioned in your interbrain and receives afferents from sensory, acute, optical and motor pathways, as well as from your spinothalamic area, your hypothalamus and your intrathalamic nuclei. It transmits information about the type and cause of stimuli to all areas of your cortex and provides the elements of cognition.

Your hypothalamus regulates sleep, metabolism, temperature, hunger, thirst and sexuality. Connected to it is your pituitary gland, which is where endocrine (hormonal) activity mainly takes place. Flight and fight reactions, the experience of fear and also the experience of other emotions, are stimulated from here. Your hypothalamus is directly connected with your reticular and thalamic system.

Your intrathalamic nuclei are the exit points of the extrapyramidal pathways. They are responsible for muscle tone, the unconscious experience of your body and automatic movements. They play an important role in your reaction to pain.

The archaic parts of your brain comprise your unconscious, susceptible part, which contains memories of your first experiences of life, as well as memories of emotional, instinctive and hormic (animalistic) experience. This is where experiences of pain are activated and where those memories are incorporated, all of which are otherwise inaccessible to your consciousness. As well as causing fear in some people, the effect of the archaic parts of the brain can also be fascinating to people, who want to discover new aspects of themselves. Your archaic brain is also the place where negative and positive conditioning occurs on an unconscious level and where it accumulates. It is accessible only to symbolic, archetypical language, which is full of imagery.

Overall, these pathways accommodate and manage your reaction to pain. Pain influences and affects all areas of your brain. In this way it stimulates potential for reaction, particularly with regard to your general health.

Neurotransmitters in labour pain

There are many chemical transmitters of pain. All nerve endings of the afferent amplifying and inhibiting pain pathways house receptors which differentiate separate chemical substances, for example the psychoactive substances somatostatin, angiotensin, neurotensin and glucagon.

While these various substances are very well-known, as yet almost nothing is understood about their precise mechanisms, which seem to follow overriding systems. The mechanism is constantly regulated and modified in response to stronger and weaker stimuli and as a result of your central evaluation of pain, which takes place in your brain. In the case of labour pain, the following neurotransmitters are particularly important...

Pain-reducing substances

Endorphins and encephalins are opiates which are produced naturally by your body. They reduce your experience of pain and instead induce a feeling of fulfilment, well-being and euphoria, as well as the desire to repeat whatever is being experienced.

These pain-reducing substances are produced in your entire nervous system, particularly in your middle brain and spinal cord, but also in your lymph cells. They are concentrated both in the gelatinous substance of your posterior horns (which are ostensibly concerned with gate control) as well as in your limbic system (which has an affective function). Nerve cells and lymph cells respond to these pain-reducing substances directly by stimulating your immune system.

The precursor of endorphins, beta-lipotropin, which is produced in your pituitary gland, is also the precursor of ACTH. There is thus an interesting connection between the build-up of ACTH, which gets dissolved when high stress and tension builds up, and the simultaneous production of endorphins, which bring a feeling of fulfilment after exertion. At the same time, ACTH can also inhibit the production of endorphins.

Serotonin and noradrenaline (a catecholamine) work to reduce the efficacy of the cells which transmit the amplifying stimuli. Serotonin is released in your brain and spinal cord. Its precise effect is not completely understood.

Pain-stimulating substances

ACTH, prostaglandins and to some extent also synthetic oxytocin (i.e. syntocinon or pitocin, which women may receive through an intravenous drip when their labour is induced or augmented) function to increase the amount of pain experienced. Any stressful situation, or contraction or over-stimulation of your sympathetic nervous system can result in the experience of pain. Oxytocin and prostaglandins are both contracting hormones. They work together in the same direction, although while prostaglandins work statically oxytocin works rhythmically. If you also experience chronic stress, the production of endorphins is inhibited. This would occur, for example, if you were induced with prostaglandins or if you were having syntocinon intravenously. Pain would then intensify and be experienced as extreme and would remain at a high level.

The compensatory mechanism for labour pain

Labour pain is very unusual because of its rhythmic nature. Due to the contrast between peaks of pain (acute stress) and absolutely painfree spaces between contractions (when there is a complete absence of noxic triggers and alarm) the production of endorphins is greatly stimulated.

This compensatory mechanism is based on the way pain develops over time. Human reproduction is well protected and is only assured when women experience birth as a fulfilling process and, consequently, want to repeat the experience. Therefore, an experience which is as painful as childbirth has to be greatly compensated for, with the help of endorphins. However, this endorphin production only occurs in the case of spontaneous births which involve no medical interventions.

A medicalised labour and birth involving synthetic (drug-based) pain relief inhibits these mechanisms and does not allow any profound fulfilment or the birthing experience which is described here. The wish to repeat the experience of giving birth is therefore dramatically reduced. As a result, we could argue a connection between the diminishing birth rate in many parts of the developed world and the lack of fulfilment women experience during unnatural labours and births.

The three neurological dimensions of pain

We need to differentiate between three basic dimensions of pain, which are always simultaneously present, but to a different extent: the sensory-perceptive, the affective-motivational and the cognitive-evaluating dimensions. These dimensions work together, each one increasing or limiting the effect of the others and, together, they are responsible for your evaluation of the pain you perceive. They influence how you experience pain during labour and how well you accept it in emotional terms. They also influence the way in which you evaluate the pain you experience and how you classify it in terms of your culture and level of knowledge.

The structures of the cerebral cortex

- The cerebral cortex is responsible for relational experience. It controls all activities in your nerve centres and can influence these either individually or all together.
- The parietal cortex performs somatosensory, associative tasks and is the exit point for a few extrapyramidal fibres.
- The temporal cortex is responsible for motor function, acute and sensitive perceptions.
- The frontal cortex includes the regions dedicated to psychomotor functions, speech centres and it is the exit point for the pyramidal pathways.
- The occipital cortex is the region governing sight and taste.

The perception, evaluation and experience of pain are influenced by central factors and these aspects of the experience are therefore highly individual. During your pregnancy, perhaps with the help of your midwife or other caregivers (e.g. a doula or a consultant), or perhaps by attending antenatal classes, you can prepare for all three dimensions of this experience.

THE SENSORY-PERCEPTIVE DIMENSION OF PAIN

This depends on conveying stimuli to your thalamus and your somato-sensory cortex. It is based in your thalamus and affects how you perceive pain. It allows you to decide where exactly it hurts, what the pain feels like and how strong it is. It determines how intensely you perceive pain and can be influenced by massage, hydrotherapy (i.e. the use of hot or cold water), warmth, coldness, compresses (hot or cold), and movement, amongst other things.

THE AFFECTIVE-MOTIVATIONAL DIMENSION OF PAIN

This dimension is affected by your limbic-reticular system. It receives stimuli from your multisynaptic system. Your reticular system is connected to all sensory and motor systems, and particularly to extrapyramidal, vegetative systems. It is responsible for all fight or flight reactions, muscular rigidity, fear, etc, as well as for vegetative reactions (which I explain overleaf).

Your limbic system reacts with a feeling of well-being or malaise, depending on the impact of the pain you experience and it consequently allows you to give pain an emotional value. The direct connection between your limbic system and your frontal cortex seems to be responsible for any unpleasant feelings which occur as a reaction to pain (Melzack, 1973).

Both these systems are receptive to influence from your neocortex and their activity can easily be altered as a result of external conditions (e.g. calmness or chaos) or from your inner sensibilities (e.g. serenity or anxiety). Depending on these factors, your reaction can be either to feel a worsening of pain or to feel more relaxed.

It seems that brain structures are activated up to a certain pain threshold (which is different for each individual woman), which promote a pleasant state of mind and interpersonal rapport. When, however, any pain exceeds this threshold, other brain structures are activated, which bring about unpleasant feelings and which create a disinclination and distancing reaction.

Overall, the affective-motivational dimension of pain influences the way you experience pain on an emotional level and it is responsible for the reaction you have to pain (for example whether you accept it, how cheerful you are, how fearful you are or how much you refuse to deal with it). During labour and birth, this dimension of pain can be positively influenced by a supportive atmosphere, by the loving closeness of your partner or a labour companion (e.g. a good friend), by positive conditions and by working on your consciousness, i.e. your state of mind.

THE COGNITIVE-EVALUATING DIMENSION OF PAIN

This dimension depends on projections of your cerebellum to your cerebral cortex and is influenced by information, cultural experiences and rationality. Your cerebral cortex receives sensory and affective information, analyses this in the light of your past experience, as well as your cultural values and your present fear, and then activates or inhibits both of the other dimensions of pain.

This process can occur selectively in your body, or throughout your whole body. If, for example, your affective-motivational system is relaxed as a result of positive experiences or a positive state of mind, you will simply recognise that pain is occurring without experiencing an unpleasant reaction, such as feeling defensive or activating your sympathetic nervous system. If, on the other hand, your system is stimulated by fear or negative cultural imprinting, then you will even experience a weak trigger as being far more painful. This dimension is the specifically human dimension of pain and therefore affects the other two dimensions.

Movement and sounds as a response to labour pain

THE MECHANISMS OF PHYSIOLOGICAL REACTIONS

First of all, there are what are called 'vegetative' reactions. These involve contractions or rigidity of your skeletal muscles and increased activity of organs which produce hormones, and of sweat glands. Your physiological reactions may involve changes in your blood pressure, heart and lung function and changes in the functioning of your internal organs.

Secondly, reactions take place in your central cerebral cortex and midbrain. These are emotional reactions, such as inner unrest and fear, and behavioural reactions determined by movement, vocalisation (for example, screaming or moaning), facial mimicry, the adoption of specific positions (which provide relief), and the immediate retreat of the part of your body which seems to be in danger (for example clamping your vagina shut).

The emotional reaction to pain is fear and tension (i.e. this is a physiological-functional reaction) or anxiety or depression. This can also be the case with chronic pain, which is dysfunctional.

The type of reaction you experience depends on the interaction of different dimensions of pain. The first two dimensions are concerned with the way in which you perceive pain, which is to do with the localisation and intensity of the pain trigger and your tendency to pull back from the pain (i.e. flee from it) or accept it. The third dimension, by contrast, is concerned with comparing the pain trigger with other triggers you have already experienced in life, which are then valued on this basis.

There are kinetic reactions in the case of both vegetative and verbal reactions to pain. When you personally experience pain you will express your own complex and highly individual reaction through your behaviour. When a midwife correctly interprets your behaviour when you're in labour, she is able to more accurately evaluate the situation which you and your unborn baby find yourselves in. The observation and correct evaluation of a labouring woman's spontaneous behaviour is one of the basic competences within the art of midwifery.

A 'CONTROLLED' REACTION TO PAIN

In some societies, even in our own, the free expression of pain experienced is not viewed positively. You may therefore feel obliged to control yourself and stay calm. If this is the case, you may consider the ideal picture of a labouring woman to be a woman who is silently biting and breathing into her handkerchief. A woman who screams or moans while she is in labour and giving birth would seem hysterical and unable to cope.

Nevertheless, when the physiological mechanisms of stimulus and response are studied it is clear that pain triggers strongly activate your affective and emotional feelings. They increase the 'electrical charge' of your feelings, as it were, and through the connections between your cerebellum and your cerebral cortex bring about a reaction to pain which takes expression in both motor and verbal respects, and in terms of neurovegetative systems. These will prompt you to move and express yourself in labour through movement and verbal expression, in an instinctual way. The expression of pain which becomes necessary on experiencing pain therefore takes the form of continual movement and instinctive behaviour, perhaps with vocalisation too (making noises).

These kinds of physiological responses to pain are powerful and liberating. Moreover, to the same extent as they have a liberating effect and reduce the electrical charge in your central nervous system, the systems which reduce levels of pain are activated and the whole effect is to minimise the overall level of pain you experience.

Sometimes the expression of labour pain is stronger than that of peripheral triggers and this will allow you to work through old memories of pain, which have remained in your subconscious. Working through labour pain therefore provides you with an opportunity to free yourself from old psychological burdens. It is not unusual for a woman to feel, after she has given birth, that she is now finally in a position to work through some old conflicts. It is also possible that a woman, who has no old pain memories to work through and who also has no previous negative experiences of childbirth, to experience no pain whatsoever, or to experience only a very small amount.

Nevertheless, we must come back to the idea of birth as a paradoxical process and once again consider physiological reactions to pain as a mechanism for enabling compensatory and transformational processes. In the case of labour pain there are two specific, mutually independent factors which make it bearable. The first is the rhythmic nature of contractions, with spaces between; the second is the build-up of endorphins which results from the experience of pain. Thanks to the rhythm of contractions, bodily reactions to pain can be changed. If, during labour, you can physically and emotionally relax in the spaces between contractions, if—during the contractions themselves—you can also take long outward breaths, if you can verbally express yourself and turn screams into singing or into open-throated tones, if you are massaged (which will help you deal with your muscular tension), if you can freely move around during contractions, if you feel so safe and protected that you can face your fear or if you simply feel free enough to uninhibitedly follow your body's needs, your reticular system will then receive no alarming messages. Instead, it will receive reassuring ones and your physiological reactions will normalise themselves and fall into an appropriate rhythm. This will make the production of endorphins possible.

In fact, during a natural, physiological birth, the verbal expression of pain usually increases and the need to move around will continue to encourage you to be active during contractions. As a result, to outside observers the pain will often seem unbearable, while in reality your actual perception of pain is reduced by all this movement and vocalisation and many women later report they mostly had feelings of overwhelming strength or of intense effort. Their pain had therefore already transmuted into something else. Therefore, instead of attempting to control pain by suppressing it, you need to allow it to be transformed. This will happen if you use your voice and move about freely!

You can help yourself in terms of the cognitive-evaluating dimension of pain during the antenatal period, particularly in antenatal classes. This means that you can prepare for this dimension well before you actually experience any labour pain. You can do this by learning about the functions of labour pain and therefore making it possible for you to become consciously motivated to work through any pain you experience. It is also important, when doing this, to collect appropriate 'weapons' for pain, so that you face it with far less fear. Read on for more information about 'weapons'.

Preparing in antenatal classes may be helpful to you

HOW THE SYMPATHETIC AND PARASYMPATHETIC SYSTEMS ARE BOTH DETECTABLE

On a psychological level, you will perceive dilation and contraction as well-being/tension-release and fear/stress; on a physical level dilation will be handled by your vagus and contraction will be handled by your sympathetic nervous system. The functions of the parasympathetic nervous system are determined by ionised potassium atoms, which is the sympathetic nervous system's calcium ionising function. Inhalation is orchestrated by the sympathetic nervous system, exhalation by the parasympathetic nervous system. If the rhythm of breathing in one direction or the other is disturbed a biological imbalance in your whole system will inevitably arise.

If your parasympathetic nervous system is more active, there will be a tendency towards expansion, opening, and tension release of your smooth muscle tissues (an activation of peristalsis). In addition, your heartbeat will slow down, your pupils will constrict, your digestion will be stimulated, you will have engorgement (hyperemia), warmth, rosy cheeks, clear eyes, your mucous membranes will be moist, you will experience positive tension and also a feeling of well-being. In this state of health your peripheral blood vessels will dilate in your genital area, your skin will pink up, and you may even expeirence feelings such as sexual arousal or ecstasy. If your heartbeat is strong and slow your labour will be easy. Your vagus therefore embodies the principle of expansion from yourself outwards, out to the whole wide world in a joyful way, just as happens in a sexual experience. (Note that this is in line with Weilhelm Reich's observations (Reich, 1942) Your sympathetic nervous system will kick into action at these moments of peak experience. At these times it will pull together your entire organism, bringing it back into balance (after extreme physical exertion) and reveal weaknesses, fear and pain.

If, on the other hand, there were insufficient blood in your uterus both your heartbeat and your breathing rate would speed up, your pupils would dilate, your lean muscle would become tense and, overall, you would feel you were in a condition of extreme clarity and alertness. In this focused and anxious (i.e. fearful) state, your peripheral blood vessels would become restricted, your skin would become pale, your mucous membranes would dry out, your heartbeat would speed up into a strained rhythm and your labour would become difficult.

The sympathetic nervous system therefore enables you to 'contract' away from the world, back into yourself (again, in line with Weilhelm Reich's observations) or it makes you experience pain and feel ill at ease. And as far as your labour would be concerned, it would have the effect of making the diagonal fibres of your uterine muscle go into spasm and hold back. Of course, this is exactly the opposite of what is necessary in the second stage of labour. The parasympathetic nervous system might override this effect if it became activated. In that case, it would have the effect of activating the long muscle fibres of the uterus and would therefore allow the second stage of labour to proceed smoothly.

The specific functions of pain in normal births

1. Pain triggers the release of hormones

Labour pain is necessary so as to ensure that you produce oxytocin, which is absolutely essential for your labour to become active. For this reason, even at the beginning of your labour (in the latent phase) it is vital that you have no drug-based forms of pain relief, because these would block your contractions.

At the beginning of your labour you will start to produce oxytocin as a result of changes in your own hormones and in those of the placenta, and also as a result of the pressure of your baby's head on your cervix. The irregular and sporadic early uterine contractions that you will experience in the latent phase are the result of this first level of oxytocin production.

In order for you to move into the active phase of labour, which is characterised by regular, contractions which effectively thin (efface) and dilate your cervix, another rhythmic stimulus needs to become activated so that your body will produce oxytocin on a constant and increasing basis. This second stimulus is *intermittent pain.*

Pain will put you into a situation of acute stress, to which your body will react in the short-term by producing a peak of stress hormones (catecholamines). Since in natural labours without drugs the production of these stress hormones occur in peaks, in a pulsatile manner, this provides the precondition (paradoxically) for increased production of oxytocin and, simultaneously, for the production of endorphins and prolactin. Energy and fatty acids will be released from cells in your body and these are precursors to prostaglandins. In this way, your labour will progress step-by-step and at the same time your pain threshold will increase.

If your body continuously produces catecholamines, for example if you experience chronic stress or if artificial oxytocics (such as syntocinon or pitocin) are pumped into your body intravenously (in a drip), your body's own production of oxytocin would be inhibited. As a result, labour would be prolonged, the latent phase would be extended and you would not move into the active stage of labour.

In many labours which do not progress beyond 3cm or 4cm dilation it has been observed that women are in a constant state of tension and at the same time they show signs of having an overstimulated sympathetic nervous system. The key in these cases would be for the woman to have her parasympathetic nervous system stimulated because this would help her find her own rhythm. She would need to use the spaces between contractions wisely. By completely relaxing between each contraction, she would be able to re-establish a state of deep calm, in which she would be free from stress and fear. If the parasympathetic nervous system were stimulated, the woman's body would then be able (during the next contraction) to produce peaks of catecholamines and thereafter also to produce the requisite amounts of oxytocin, which would both help her labour progress. Therefore, when you're in labour if you yourself find that you are in a state of chronic stress and tension first of all you would need to stop yourself from having contractions by stimulating your parasympathetic system. Only when you were in a state of deep relaxation would the contractions be able to spontaneously re-establish themselves in a physiological rhythm. A good way of stimulating your parasympathetic nervous system is to use Polarity Therapy (see Chapter 6), as well as massage and relaxation techniques, such as singing, visualisation and similar activities. (Obviously, you need to get a birth partner involved with some of these!)

The harmonious cooperation of both parts of the nervous system is extremely important during childbirth because both parts are responsible for orchestrating contractions. While your sympathetic nervous system gives you *strength,* your parasympathetic nervous system will help the lower segment of your uterus and your cervix to open up. If both systems do not work together in harmony you would experience:

- ineffective contractions without dilation
- lack of coordination between your uterus and cervix or vaginal tone (indicating dominance of your sympathetic nervous system
- uterine hypotonia, i.e. over-exertion, with so-called 'passive dilation' which would be inadequate for progress in labour and the second stage to occur successfully (which requires dominance of the parasympathetic nervous system)

Make sure you relax in the spaces between contractions

In other words, the harmonious working of both systems is facilitated by the rhythm of contractions and through relaxation in the spaces between them. You can do a great deal to help promote the harmony of this process by relaxing in the spaces between contractions and by focusing on discovering your own inner resources for coping with pain. You can quickly reach a state of deep relaxation, if you give yourself up to the contractions. This state will mean that physiological pain is reduced to an absolute minimum.

Another important aspect of pain as an endocrine stimulator concerns the production of endorphins. The task of endorphins is not exclusively to limit your experience of pain. During the first stage of your labour endorphins will also bring about a change in your state of consciousness... you will go into a kind of trance, or into a spontaneous state of hypnosis. In doing so, the rational side of your mind, the neocortex, will be inhibited and this will in turn support the functioning parts of your brain (your cerebellum and your autonomic nervous system). This will enable your labour to progress in an optimal way and it will make it possible for you to completely give yourself up to the natural processes. This will then lead to a full opening up, so that you are able to separate yourself from your baby and joyfully welcome it into this world.

If you fully open up, you can separate from your baby

At the moment of your baby's birth, when contractions suddenly stop, there are extremely high levels of endorphins in your body (after an unmedicated, physiological labour) and these will make you feel very satisfied about your own achievement, and also make you feel ecstatic and euphoric. These are the feelings you will experience when you first meet your new baby and when you begin your experience as a mother.

We can also attribute feelings of dependency and attachment to endorphins. Bonding is of course the most important precondition for the baby to live and indeed thrive. We can therefore say that a natural, physiological birth gives the baby an excellent start in life.

In order to facilitate the process of separation of yourself from your baby (during the birth)—to make it easier for your baby to separate from you—ironically enough, you need to build a good connection with your baby throughout your pregnancy. Have an inner dialogue with your baby and thereby put your baby at centre stage during your labour, so that your baby will seem more real to you and less alien, and so that it does not only exist in your imagination. The better communication is between you and your baby, the more easily the process of separation at birth will flow. This will mean that the birth itself will take place more quickly and smoothly and will mean that you experience less pain.

2. Pain leads you through birth and protects you and your baby

It is often the physiological task of pain to protect your body from injury. In cases of attack it provides an 'alarm signal' and thereby helps you to quickly take appropriate action so as to distance yourself from danger. For example, pain makes you pull a burnt finger out of the fire. In this and many other cases, pain therefore functions to make you active.

During the birth, the opening up of muscles which are usually closed (particularly your cervix and perineum) and which usually protect your body, and the strong pressure on your sacroiliac joint and nerves in that area of your body caused by your descending baby's head present some risk for both you and your baby. Pain therefore functions as a valuable guide because it shows you danger and puts you in a position where you can change your situation by the way in which you behave. Your inevitable physiological reaction to pain will be *movement*. When it is not possible for you to move spontaneously, without inhibition, the experience of pain becomes a form of martyrdom and cannot be justified.

Freedom of movement during labour allows you to instinctively find positions which make your pain more bearable. These are also the positions which will provide the least amount of pressure and resistance for your baby's head, which allow it to be eased out of your body. These positions also reduce your baby's stress, so prevent asphyxia (i.e. oxygen deprivation).

If you are free to move you will experience less pain

As you protect yourself from damage to your pelvis, cervix and perineum (by moving around) you also will protect your unborn baby from malpositioning and unnecessary pressure on its head. As a result, you will minimise the risk of fetal distress and the risk of oxygen deficiency (asphyxia). At the same time, the pain you experience will stimulate the production of endorphins, which exist in the highest concentrations in the amniotic fluid. Of course, this means that your unborn baby will also be protected from pain and trauma.

Often, during labour, you will only be able to tolerate very specific positions, sometimes precisely those which seemed the least probable to you during antenatal courses or in your pregnancy generally—because labour pain is very specific in its instructions! In this way, pain will lead you through your labour, showing you how to behave appropriately. By providing you with physical sensations, it will also help you to feel a sense of what to do at whichever stage of labour and birth you find yourself.

3. Pain facilitates your baby's descent and facilitates the birth

This function of pain is clearly connected with the psychological side of labour as well as the physical side.

During labour, one of the most intense feelings women experience is the feeling that they must 'get free of the baby'. In other words, they feel a deep need to separate themselves from their baby, which is simultaneously part of themselves and also a being in its own right, which lives in both the woman's imagination and her fantasies, as well as in the real world. The way in which you will experience this need to separate will also determine how your baby will find its way through your pelvis and how long this will take.

Separating from something that has become part of you or from somebody who you have become very close to is always painful, difficult and often also involuntary. In the case of childbirth it is both an event which is longed for and feared. Your newborn baby may seem foreign to you and he or she may make you a little fearful, or you may accept him or her confidently, with joy.

In fact, pain will function to lead you inescapably in the direction of separation—a direction which you might take voluntarily. Pain will make it clear to you that birth is unavoidable and necessary and it will concentrate all your attention on this process, leaving you no escape route beyond actually coming to grips with the task of giving birth. At the same time, the pain you experience will in itself be an expression and outlet for the emotional suffering, which separation inevitably involves.

Pain will determine the pace... and the timing of this separation process is an important factor, which varies considerably from person to person. The more intense the contractions you experience, the faster the separation will take place. If the intensity of pain is reduced (through the use of drug-based pain relief) your need to separate from your baby will seem less urgent and so the process may take longer.

Risks associated with restricting your movements during labour

Positions for labour and birth are still, as ever, being determined in too many cases by the protocols and traditions of a maternity unit or birthing centre. This is the case just as much for normal, spontaneous births as it is for births which involve medico-technical support.

In the first stage of labour you are most likely to be given freedom of movement, but you may be limited because of the 'necessity' for electronic fetal monitoring (EFM). (In fact, EFM is unnecessary in normal labours—intermittent monitoring of the fetal heartbeat with a fetoscope (Pinard) or Sonicaid is perfectly adequate.) During this first stage of labour women are often asked to lie down in bed, and this may even be insisted upon, even in many hospitals in Britain, France and Germany, not to mention the USA and elsewhere. Lying down is often disguised as being a 'half-sitting' position on a hospital bed. If your movements are limited in this way there are numerous disadvantages for both you and your baby.

Risks if you labour and give birth lying down—for you

- Painful and less effective contractions, which would not allow you to position yourself appropriately in terms of your birth canal
- Significantly less relaxation in the spaces between contractions since the lower segment of your uterus would remain tense
- Longer 'peaks' in contractions and consequently more pressure on the tissues (in your pelvis), resulting in more pain
- An increased risk of cervical injury
- Extreme pressure on your sacroiliac joint and on your coccyx (tailbone), which might lead to long-term back pain or damage to your coccyx
- A more probable need for artificial oxytocics (i.e. a drip) and other drugs
- Increased pressure on your vena cava (vena-cava compression syndrome), which could mean poor blood flow from your placenta and inadequate blood flow to your heart; as a result, low blood pressure could result which would need to be dealt with or monitored carefully
- The lack of an opportunity to spontaneously recognise the urge to push and your consequent inability to respond to this; this could well lead to extreme exertion, exhaustion and could also cause some caregivers (outside the UK) to use fundal pressure so as to make the birth possible; the risks associated with applying fundal pressure from your point of view are: uterine prolapse, rib fractures, extreme retinal or ocular pressure, broken blood vessels in your face, cervical tears, vaginal tears, perineal tears, premature placental abruption and uterine rupture (all bad news!)
- Perineal tears and frequent episiotomy (since pressure on the perineum would be significantly greater if you were lying down, compared to if you were in an upright position); both tears and episiotomy would increase the risk of infection, haemorrhage and other after-effects, they would make bonding more difficult (since suturing would need to take place straight after the birth, when you should really be bonding with your newborn baby) ... and they would also increase the likelihood that you would have difficulty breastfeeding

Risks if you labour and give birth lying down—for your baby

- An increased likelihood of fetal distress (as a result of a lack of oxygen) because of longer contraction peaks
- Decreased oxygen availability in the spaces between contractions since you would be less relaxed
- Increased pressure on your baby's head, since babies who are born of mothers who are lying down are three times more likely to suffer from convulsions in their first year of life than babies born of mothers who were able to freely choose their position for giving birth (Paciornik, 1982)
- Increased likelihood of variable fetal heart decelerations and meconium-stained amniotic fluid and consequently an increased risk of a caesarean section
- More frequent malpositioning of the fetal head in the second stage of labour as a result of forced pushing (with you holding your breath), either as a result of compression of the vena cava or as a result of fundal pressure
- Extreme pressure on your unborn baby's head in the second stage of labour
- Increased likelihood of umbilical cord entanglement
- More frequent need for resuscitation of your newborn baby and consequent separation of your baby from you, meaning a later first feed and delayed bonding

Lying down involves all kinds of risks for your baby

The connection between pain and sexuality in childbirth

According to Wilhelm Reich[18] the ability to reach orgasm is the ability to give oneself up to the flow of biological energy without inhibition and replace the sexual tension which has built up with involuntary contractions.

Considering the experience of birth we could say that the ability to give birth is the ability to give oneself up to the flow of biological energy without inhibition and without resistance and to replace accumulated tension with radiating, rhythmical, involuntary contractions.

The enormous strength involved in giving birth—which is little known and little understood, but greatly feared—means that for you childbirth is a powerful expression of your quintessential femininity, as well as an expression of that aspect of your sexuality which is independent from men.

If you wish, you can also share this experience with your partner. If you give birth to your baby through the power of your own sexuality you will have a more intense feeling of womanhood after the birth. In every respect you will feel strengthened, but particularly in the sense of your orgasmic ability, which Wilhelm Reich wrote about.

The means of experiencing this orgasm-like experience during labour and birth is not a feeling of well-being but rhythmic pain. With ongoing, increasing arousal tension increases in your body, particularly in the area of your genitals .

As a result of your body's increasing production of endorphins you become increasingly capable of letting yourself go to the flow of biological energy, you become more and more relaxed, you let yourself go completely and you move into a different state of consciousness.

When the tension caused by pain has reached a certain level, in the spaces between contractions your body prepares you to release this tension through 'involuntary rhythmic contractions'—first through your whole body (which may produce shivering and a feeling of coldness), then through your pelvic floor muscles (where you will feel involuntary pressure). The pressure of your baby's head in your vagina will be the final stimulus which will allow you to release cumulative tension through involuntary contractions and allow your baby to cross your pelvic floor and—with long out-breaths—give birth to your baby.

After this, energy which has become concentrated in the area of your genitals will flow back through your entire body. You will experience this as a return of strength, a sense of fulfilment and a feeling of well-being. These feelings also will express themselves in the form of tenderness and gratitude during the immediate postnatal bonding stage, in the first hours after you have given birth.

If you can give birth to your baby and accept it, experiencing pain and consequently the strength of your sexual energy, if you can release your own tension through the birth itself and regain your energy after the birth, you will not feel either shivery or cold afterwards... you will only feel a sense of satisfaction and complete tenderness.

If you understand birth in this way, then you will naturally see your partner as being much more than that of a 'patient spectator' during your labour. Moreover, it you will be able to see that both you and your partner together will have an ever-increasing need (during your labour and the birth itself) for intimacy, making the situation comparable to the requirements needed for undisturbed lovemaking.

Just as instructions about breathing, movement, eye contact and the use of your mouth would be of little use to you just before an orgasm, this kind of interference would only inhibit the progress of your birthing experience during the second stage of labour.

Things which increase the pain of labour and birth

- Muscular tension
- Cervical scars or irritation
- Tension in the lower segment of your uterus
- Hypertonia in your cervix (as a result of the use of synthetic oxytocin or increased muscular resistance)
- A low pain threshold
- Adhesions in your pelvis or ovaries
- Lack of freedom of movement
- Unnatural physical positioning (e.g. lying down with your legs up in stirrups, lying down generally or a retroverted—tilted back—pelvis)

- Tension and fear
- Negative expectations of labour pain
- Negative previous personal experience, or hearing about other women's negative experiences
- Lack of any bonding with your growing baby during pregnancy
- Stimulation of your neocortex (through bright light, open doors, etc) and a foreign-feeling environment
- Interventions without your agreement
- Passivity and a tendency to delegate responsibility
- The lack of any human support
- The lack of any recovery during spaces between contractions
- The medicalisation of birth through the use of intravenous drips, amniotomy (having your waters broken), manual stretching the cervix, commanded pushing or in-labour encouragement, the non-acceptance of personal needs, episiotomy (a large cut in your perineum), etc
- The early separation of you and your newborn baby soon after the birth

Things which reduce the pain of labour and birth

- A mobile pelvis
- Good pelvic floor elasticity and the ability to tense or relax pelvic muscles
- A soft, effaced and centralised cervix towards the end of your pregnancy
- Normal uterine tone
- A high pain threshold
- Freedom of movement
- The freedom to behave as you wish (instinctively) and vocalise uninhibitedly
- Postures which include an anteverted, open pelvis
- Respect of individual rhythms
- Trust and acceptance of labour pain, with an understanding of its purpose
- Motivation and realistic expectations of pain
- A calming and intimate atmosphere
- Support from your partner or another well-known person
- Good contact between you and your baby, even during pregnancy
- Conservative, protective and respectful care (i.e. watchful waiting, while your midwife or consultant creates an atmosphere of safety and respect)
- Professional support and sensitive midwifery care
- A warm bath
- Deep relaxation in the spaces between contractions
- An unforced second stage, with spontaneous, involuntary pushing contractions
- An intact perineum
- Undisturbed early contact with your newborn baby (to facilitate bonding), especially in the first hours after the birth

The psychological, emotional and spiritual meaning of pain

Pain can be a component of your personal development. Every baby who is born enables its mother to have a new experience. Every birth is different—unique—and holds within it special potential for your own development.

Nevertheless, the first birth you experience will have a stronger meaning for you than subsequent births. This is because the first time you give birth you are encountering something entirely unknown, which will alter your status. After this experience of birth you will no longer be first and foremost your mother's daughter, but the mother of a child.

The energy potential of a profound inner transformation lies in the uniqueness of the biological situation, in which you will find yourself while you are in labour and giving birth. At no other moment in your life will you produce such incredibly high levels of hormones. The hormones will strongly stimulate your hypothalamus and they will act as neurotransmitters. As a result, they will have a great impact on your feelings and instincts and will serve to inform all the cells in your body about what is happening. As has already been explained, the hormones of birth will put you in a trance-like state, which will constitute a change in consciousness (which will be identifiable by the observation of alpha and theta brainwaves). The slower your brainwaves are, the more likely it is that you will experience a feeling of oneness, integration and spiritual understanding. Simply as a result of pregnancy, your brainwaves will slow down and this process will be facilitated through breathing, relaxation, meditation and contemplation, massage and the production of endorphins. From what is already known about brain waves and the development of the baby's brain, we can deduce that your growing baby will experience theta waves exclusively in the first half of your pregnancy and alpha waves later on (Hannaford, 2008).

When you give birth you can be directly connected both to your baby and also to the energies in the universe, if you tune your consciousness into your biological experience. In this sense, birth can take on a distinctly spiritual character, which can extend your world view.

Another aspect of personal development stems from the battle you may have with your own resources, which will probably force you to go beyond your own normal limits of experience. Facing unfamiliar pain creates fear and anxiety; having to work with this pain for hours on end will put your strength to the test. It is therefore possible to say that pain is likely to trigger a real existential crisis, which will mobilise all your emotions, including old 'fire' (deep wounds, injuries, past pain), from the depths of your subconscious, and this will all bring you to the very edges of your ability to cope.

At the point where you feel you have exhausted all your resources, you will come to a point of capitulation. You may well shout out, 'But I just can't go on!'—and doing this will involve total surrender, which will in turn allow your active body to flow with powerful energies. Surrendering like this will mean going beyond your own normal limits and activating strong new resources i.e. it will mean a transformation. You will then give birth, you will bring another person into the world and in doing so you will add to your own personal strength.

The growth in personal strength which occurs as a result of going beyond the normal boundaries of experience signifies (even in the case of difficult births) that a necessary maturation process has taken place. This, in turn, gives a woman the strength she needs in order to be able to take good care of her baby and bring it up properly.

The influence of contractions on your baby while it is being born

One of the most striking things about a newborn is its ability to mimic facial expressions and thereby communicate. It is enough to observe a newborn baby when it emerges out of its mother's vulva to understand what it has just experienced. Some babies are born with obvious physical signs of discomfort or distress and some are not. We need to consider what might affect the experience of a newborn baby.

Birth is an event which is strongly determined by the quality of communication between you and your baby. The functional harmony between dynamic and mechanical factors depends directly on this communication, which explains the synchrony of head moulding and cervical dilation. Therefore, the better the flow of communication and consciousness between you and your baby, the more naturally and instinctually your labour and birth will proceed. In addition, the fewer traumatic interventions that take place (such as amniotomy, augmentation of labour with artificial oxytocin, manual cervical stretching, fundal pressure and other interventions which aim to speed up the birthing process), the less your baby will suffer.

When contact between you and your baby is difficult your resistance to the opening process of birth would easily increase so that birth would become a kind of battle between someone who wants to 'be born' (i.e. your baby) and someone who doesn't want to 'die' or give up (i.e. you!). When, on the other hand, a baby is too little involved in its birth, it withdraws, making interventions necessary. In both cases, the baby's suffering increases.

When labour pain is reduced to a minimum it becomes bearable for both mother and baby. As a result of the high levels of endorphins which are present in the amniotic fluid your baby will be well protected. Of course, these endorphins will increase greatly when you produce them yourself by experiencing pain. In other words, if you experience pain you will actually *protect* your baby from pain.

Contractions your labour will be important for your baby because the normal pressure on his or her head in the birth canal, which these contractions will cause, will enable your baby to produce fetal adrenaline. This is a hormone which is essential for adaptation to life outside the womb and which will protect your baby from asphyxiation (i.e. breathing difficulties). Nevertheless, if pressure on your baby's head were to be too strong because of malpresentation or interventions, this would mean pain for your baby postnatally. (This explains why it would not be helpful for contractions to be artificially accelerated with artificial oxytocin.)

The rhythm between contractions and spaces between contractions will prepare your newborn baby for breathing (which will have the same cyclical rhythm), and also for the contrasts on which all human experience is based. Through the production of adrenaline, the pain of your labour will make your newborn baby strong and capable of fighting, so that he or she will be able to take hold of his or her own life.

Without the rhythm of labour, either because you are unable to relax fully in the spaces between contractions, or because you are very fearful so remain continuously tense, your baby would probably suffer more. The risk of asphyxiation would increase for your newborn baby, its level of catecholamines would increase and the level of endorphins would decline. In other words, if you were to have a difficult, obstructed birth, your baby would share your suffering. If, on the other hand, you have a natural, instinctive and flowing birth, your baby is unlikely to suffer.

In this and all the other ways we have discussed in this chapter, the physiology of labour and birth serves many important functions. When the physiological processes are changed through the use of drug-based pain relief, it is not possible for labour to function in the same ways. Labour and birth then become a very different experience for both mother and baby and even more drug-based intervention is required (usually along with many obstetric interventions) because, in fact, neither physical nor psychological pain relief is achieved, as was hoped. When the natural processes are disturbed in that way, the whole experience of birth is more likely to be a trauma to be endured, rather than a process which can be transformational for you, and health-promoting for your baby.

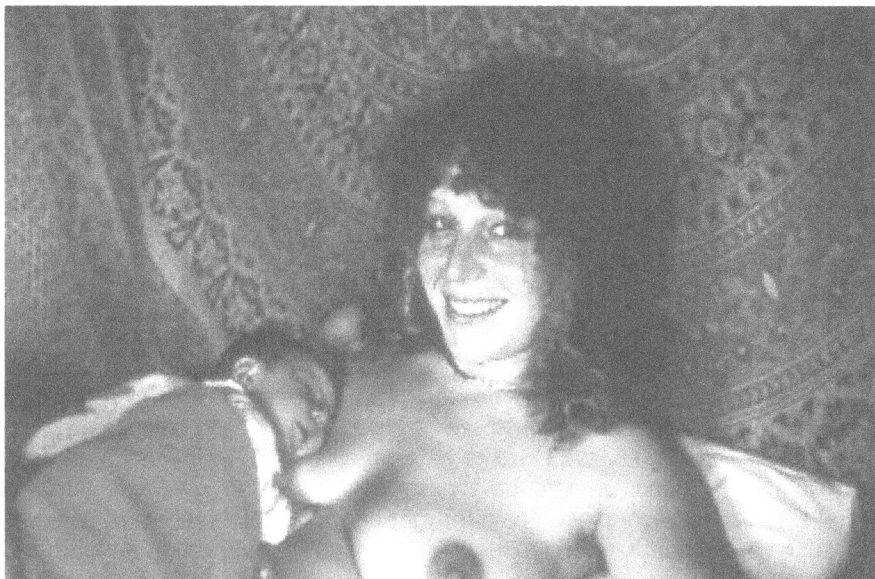

A new mother, soon after giving birth, without any drugs or interventions

CHAPTER 3:

Elective caesareans—
the supposedly simpler alternative

Why do some women want a caesarean?

In order to answer this question, we should really ask each individual woman who has requested an elective caesarean why she wants to bring her child into the world in this way. Reasons are certainly integrally connected to each woman's personal history and are therefore very individual. Nevertheless, at this point I must make some generalisations in order to shed light on this area.

I shall start from the perspective of physiology. What occurs during the birthing process? Childbirth essentially involves a physical and spiritual opening up of one's being, which is in conflict with any woman's instinct for self-preservation. The total opening up which birth involves creates fear, because it goes against a woman's natural instinct for self-protection.

Bodily processes which are normally controlled consciously by the left-hand side of the brain change quite dramatically during pregnancy and birth. The right-hand side of the brain takes over and the balance between the two sides of the brain gradually disappears. Feelings and instincts, which up until this time had lain dormant in the subconscious, rise to the surface. Hormonal production increases dramatically and forces the mother-to-be into a situation from which only birth itself can save her (Davis, 2000).

During this process, I would suggest that the body feels itself to be existentially threatened and physiologically that it experiences the process as an attack because the baby within is making inroads into the mother's physical integrity. From a physiological point of view, childbirth can therefore be seen as an act of aggression, but it also has a paradoxical status in that it is integrally concerned with the preservation of the species.

In order to deal with the potential threat that birth involves, the fight-flight response is strongly activated in the woman. On the one hand the body reacts to the danger signals it perceives, but on the other hand the body fulfils its purpose, which is to preserve the species.

FUNCTIONS OF THE FIGHT-FLIGHT RESPONSE

Your flight-flight adaptation response is directed by your archaic brain (your hypothalamus, pituitary gland, thalamus and your limbic system), by your sympathetic nervous system and by your adrenal glands.

In order to deal with the threat that birth involves, the fight-flight response is strongly activated in the woman

First, an internal or external event reaches your archaic brain and puts it into a state of alert. Your sympathetic nervous system then prepares your body to respond instinctively (through the production of adrenaline), it brings blood to your muscles, activates your adrenal glands to produce hormones (catecholamines, cortisol) and provides you with a boost of energy.

As a result of this process there is an instinctive response to restore a state of safety which involves either 'flight' (in order to take you away from the danger), or 'fight' (in order to deal with the threat). The explosion of some kind of physical action then allows your body to return to a state of rest. When no instinctive behaviour follows, the explosive reaction remains hidden in your body and leads to distress.

Giving birth constitutes the only possible way for you to distance yourself from the potential threat you may perceive. You would therefore have to decide on 'flight' if you didn't want to give birth.

'Flight' would lead inevitably to withdrawal, closing yourself off, distress, dystocia, an epidural or a caesarean. Sometimes behaviour associated with 'flight' might agitate you to the point where you find it impossible to 'fight' (i.e. to give birth). In this case, still within the fight-flight metaphor, 'fighting' is only possible when you—the 'woman in battle'— own special weapons and when you are sure of yourself. You would need to be familiar with the 'danger' in order to face it effectively and you would need to be strongly motivated to do so.

'Fight' in the female sense also means surrender, letting yourself go. Paradoxically, during childbirth 'fight' for you will mean facing the danger by opening up to your baby within and gaining distance from the danger by letting your baby go free. The hormonal answer to the stress of birth is not adrenaline but oxytocin and prolactin. These lead to a 'tend and befriend reaction' (Taylor, 2002).

It is important that you behave instinctively for this to be possible. Only by using your intuition, which can assess the situation on a moment-by-moment basis, can you activate the appropriate, focused, unconscious impulses you need in order to give birth. You must listen to your intuition and take it seriously. And in preparation for your labour and birth you need to create a special environment with sufficient intimacy for the birth and thereby activate your parasympathetic nervous system (i.e. the right-hand side of your brain). Only then can you 'open yourself up'.

What does it mean to 'open yourself up'?

'Opening yourself up' means making yourself vulnerable, going deep inside yourself and into the darkness, confronting your subconscious. It means allowing yourself to feel and to express yourself freely. It means coming into contact with the essence of your being. It means letting your feelings rise to the surface and losing rational control, although not losing touch with yourself and not losing awareness of your bodily sensations.

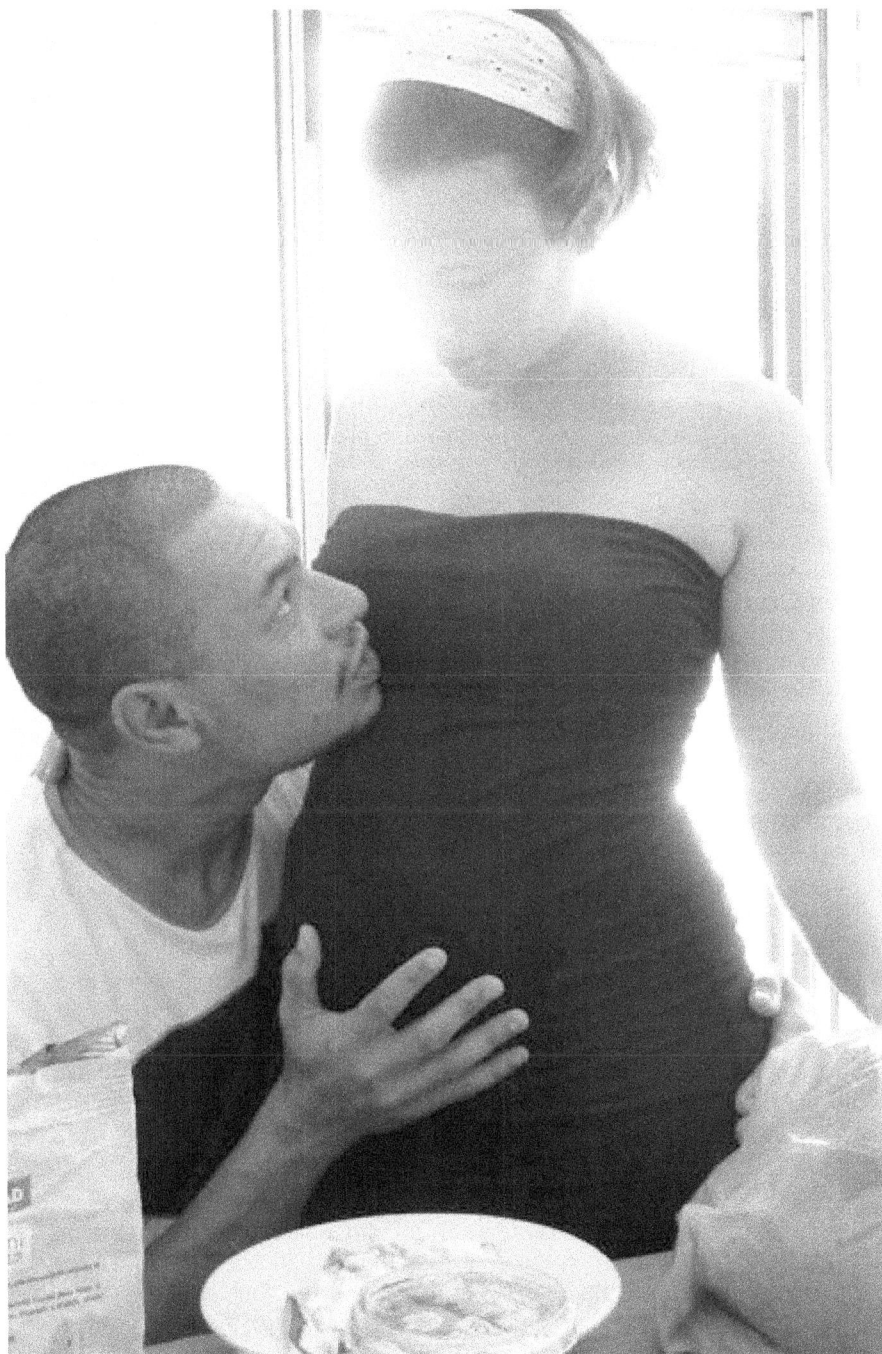

The prospect of a vaginal birth might be frightening for both you and your partner

The prospect of opening up may make you feel more fear than pain. In order to allow yourself to have this experience you need to have a totally protected space. It will then be possible for you to have a deep sexual experience and make contact with old, archaic, archetypical wisdom. If you do this an enormous resource emerges—a source of strength to carry on living.

In our society, with our contemporary lifestyle, there is no room for these kinds of processes and we avoid them, where possible. 'Control' is the name of the game!—and the simplest, cleanest and most predictable form of control over birth events takes the form of a caesarean section: a surgical opening made under narcotic trance, which requires no active participation and which dredges up no deep feelings. The technological paradox is a birth under epidural anaesthesia taking place in front of a blaring television, which requires no focus on the events of birth, on the baby... This kind of birth represents total alienation from the physical and psychosexual processes.

The technological model of birth

Within a technological model of birth both pregnancy and birth are medicalised because a woman's body is seen as being unpredictable, so it must therefore, be kept under constant control. Everything is seen as involving 'risk' and this results in a great deal of fear. Even the baby is seen as being part of this risk-paradigm, and is supposedly in constant danger, so machines are seen as being better at watching over the fetus or baby than its own mother.

Although you are still capable of tuning into a known and real danger when you are pregnant, and behaving appropriately with your fight-or-flight response, you may well become confused when presented with abstract threats and you may therefore move into a state of distress, which may be linked with feelings of fear and inadequacy.

Furthermore, the technological model of birth communicates to you that pain and feelings are unnecessary, that birth does not necessarily involve ecstasy and fulfilment. It communicates that bonding with your baby is not a significant theme associated with birth since you do, after all, have your cultural capabilities as a human being. The traditional 'animal' way of birthing babies, through a vagina, no longer fits into our rational, progressive culture. Non-medical birth attendants are not required and many women who still give birth vaginally are at the mercy of both pain from unnatural birthing conditions and medical interventions. You may therefore find yourself listening to many fear-inducing reports of birth.

While many midwives try to support and empower women, the obstetric model of birth responds to these fears by offering epidurals and caesareans. In no way is concern for women the only thing that is significant here... Economic factors as well as a patriarchal system of power are just as important. This system wants to control and dominate you and your potential for reproduction, and direct the event of 'childbirth' from the left-hand side of your brain. In this system the essence of birth is not understood, because the cyclical nature of life-death-life is not recognised.

From a medical point of view elective caesareans are promoted and respected along with any other female request. It is a 'doctor-friendly' choice, though. Within this paradigm of 'choice' is concealed the drive to squeeze the events of your birth into a rational framework, which is less threatening to your caregivers. The denial of death is an additional factor, which makes elective caesareans politically and medically legitimate, despite the well-documented side-effects of caesarean sections, which include a higher maternal mortality rate (Donati, *et al*, 2001).

Within the paradigm of 'choice' is concealed the drive to squeeze the events of birth into a rational framework

The dismembered woman

For the same reasons, woman has been 'dismembered' over the centuries. The control of womankind has gone beyond her body and has also left behind traces in her soul. Not only during childbirth but also in other sensitive phases of a woman's life do injuries take place, which leave behind scars, negative conditioning and a tendency to run away from events. As a result, if you have experienced mistreatment, rape or sexual abuse (for example), you may find it extremely difficult to surrender to the opening up processes of birth.

In 1977 at the peak of obstetric development in medicine, a stone was found in Mexico City, which shows Coyolxauhqui, the dismembered goddess of the moon. She symbolises the disturbance and rebirth of the feminine element. Dismembered goddesses also exist in other cultures. They represent the disturbance of female values, cutting and separation—all of which are central in male systems of values. However, these goddesses also represent rebirth, which inevitably follows on from dismemberment.

Modern obstetrics can therefore be seen to represent the continuation of the historical dismemberment which has taken place, as well as—in some cases—liberation for the dismembered woman, which takes the form of the caesarean operation. Women who believe in the power of their own bodies should be looking for other forms of resolution.

What do women really choose?

In Brazil women choose to have a caesarean in order to keep their sexual organs intact. Do they not know that a natural birth can be orgasmic, that sexual experience becomes more profound as a result and that the sensitivity of the vagina can become strengthened as a result of a vaginal birth?

In Italy women have told me they opt for a caesarean in order to avoid inhumane maternity care. Do they not know about other possibilities for birth?

Women opt for a caesarean so as to avoid inhumane care

Women may choose a caesarean to avoid facing feelings

In Britain women may choose to have a caesarean in order to sidestep deep feelings and pain, to determine the day of the birth themselves or because they see it as a lifestyle choice. Do they not know about the emotional connection they could have with their baby, which would promote its mental and spiritual growth? Do you personally have any reasons for wanting to avoid birth?

The popularity of VBAC (vaginal birth after caesarean) suggests that many women choose not to have another caesarean after a first caesarean. Most women seem to want to have a spontaneous birth the second time round. Women who opt for an elective caesarean for the birth of a subsequent child after a first vaginal birth are mostly women who have had a traumatic birth, involving drug-based pain relief, epidurals, episiotomy, etc. Behind the supposedly self-determined choice for a caesarean there is therefore fear, over-medicalisation and disorientation, all of which may come as a result of media influence and conflicts of power.

Short- and long-term effects of caesareans

HEALTH-RELATED EFFECTS

When caesareans are performed maternal mortality increases approximately four-fold compared to spontaneous vaginal delivery. Haemorrhage, infections, pulmonary embolism and bladder injury are possible short-term complications, as well as complications arising as a result of the use of anaesthesia. Transfusions, anaemia, slow healing of wounds, endometriosis, pelvic abscesses or thrombophlebitis and fever are all potential problems postnatally. Longer hospital stays, postpartum pain, depression and breastfeeding problems are also common consequences of a caesarean (Wagner, 2001). There are also possible long-term consequences, such as placental problems in subsequent pregnancies, increased frequency of ectopic pregnancy, hysterectomy and decreased fertility or sterility (Wagner, 2000).

For the baby various complications are possible, quite apart from the risk of scalpel injuries. For example, the baby may well have problems adapting to the external environment, since a planned caesarean usually means a birth which is too early from the baby's point of view, so it is not yet ready. Since the baby experiences no contractions it also produces no fetal adrenaline and as a result it is not prepared for the changed environment outside the womb. This means it often experiences difficulties with breathing and temperature regulation (since it is not able to use its brown fat). It also often has trouble orienting itself during the first feed and while meeting its mother for the first time. (The baby does not take the initiative itself, as happens after an unmedicated vaginal birth.) After a caesarean the baby also retains less placental blood and therefore has a higher risk of anaemia in its first year of life. A further well-documented long-term complication of caesareans is asthma (Mercer, *et al,* 2007).

BEHAVIOURAL EFFECTS

After a caesarean a woman's freedom of movement is severely limited during the first few days after the birth as a result of postoperative pain and over the next six to eight weeks this continues because of decreased abdominal muscle control. The mother's relationship with her baby is consequently affected, along with breastfeeding and the general postnatal atmosphere. A dysphoric (depressed) mother—one who is experiencing the opposite of euphoria will negatively affect her baby's natural tendency to suckle at the breast.

EFFECTS ON FEELINGS

The effects caesareans have on feelings are strong but rarely noted. After a caesarean women report feeling exposed and helpless. They feel they have been cheated of their birth experience; they feel a lack of fulfilment; they report psychological, more than physical pain, decreased self-esteem and feelings of helplessness. And their wish to have further children is significantly reduced. Furthermore, the whole physical and psychological mother-baby relationship is shaped by the caesarean experience.

The effects caesareans have on feelings are rarely noted

What does a baby experience when it's born by caesarean?

Nadia Filippini, a Venetian historian (Filippini, 1995), calls the caesarean section 'birth without a mother'. The child is in indeed born, but it isn't welcomed properly by a woman who has been transformed into a mother—so it's not born to its mother. In the case of an elective caesarean the baby is alone and unprepared postnatally. I would imagine it cannot understand what is happening and reacts with a feeling of disorientation. What I think must be missing is the feeling of strength it would normally experience and the ability to react to the external environment. Because the baby made no decision (to be born) it can't be aware of its own birth as it would normally be. The way a birth takes place is important for the separation of the child and unconditional opening-up helps the woman transform herself into a mother. It also helps her to receive her new baby appropriately.

Since there is a lack of adrenaline in a caesarean birth, children born in this way are significantly more susceptible to stress. It is more difficult for them to adapt to the outside world and they have difficulty becoming oriented. According to Michel Odent, caesarean-born babies lack the biological language of love because they have been born without the hormones of love, i.e. oxytocin, endorphins and prolactin (Taylor, 2002). Nowadays, the question as to how to prevent violence is a hot topic of discussion... perhaps this lack of natural oxytocin and prolactin, the hormone of protection at the time of birth, should also be taken into account.

The impact on the biological process of becoming a woman

Pregnancy, birth and the first year of life follow biologically determined rhythms, all of which aim to help your baby adapt to his or her new life. These rhythms, which were established during pregnancy, will repeat themselves and become even stronger during the first year of life within your relationship with your child. By the end of this period, you will have learnt these rhythms. Seen from a biological point of view, these rhythms are determined by the hormones your baby produces, but are modulated by your and your baby's behaviour and feelings when you interact. The basic rhythm of pregnancy and birth is as follows:

- **First trimester** You adapt as a result of experiencing crises and fears.
- **Second trimester** A kind of integration takes place because you and your baby develop a symbiotic relationship. You opens yourself up and you actively maintain your equilibrium.
- **Third trimester** You feel excited and begin to separate yourself from your baby by nesting. You switch from active to passive increasingly often and therefore become ready for the rhythm of contractions. You experience an increase in energy and tension and your fight-or-flight response system becomes activated.

During the birth itself these themes are repeated:

- Early labour corresponds to what is happening in the first trimester.
- The active stage of labour (when contractions are coming thick and fast) mirrors the opening process occurring during the second trimester.
- The second stage of labour (the birth) is similar to the third trimester.

Then, as soon as your child is born, this cycle begins again. The rhythm characterised by bonding and separation repeats itself again and again as your child grows up. Bonding is a pre-condition for your ability to separate and is necessary for individual development.

As we have seen, both birth and preparation for birth are missing in the case of an elective caesarean. It is also important to note other missing elements: the usual pre-birth burst of energy, the opening-up process (so that it is possible for you to separate yourself from your baby) and afterwards the action of taking your baby back again (so you can look after him or her). The energy of pregnancy cannot be offloaded so easily. If you were to have an unnecessary, non-medically indicated caesarean your flight-or-flight response would be replaced by a kind of paralysis: you would be kept within your own limits and you would have no access to your own resources. Your ability to be aggressive, to fight instinctively, would get lost, you would become static and you would lose your strength and power and, most importantly, you would no longer have a choice because other people would make decisions for you. And when your baby arrived, torn from your body without the biological help of hormones and without the humane help of wise midwives, you would feel helpless and unprepared, faced with your baby and his or her demands. Pain, fears, deep feelings and difficulties, all of which you wanted to avoid by having an elective caesarean, might well appear repeatedly and might be particularly strong after the birth of your first child.

Can elective caesareans be ethically justified?

If we look at the scientific evidence and the quality of the birth experience, should caregivers really allow women to choose an intervention which damages their health and increases their risk of dying? Given the evidence, how can the ethics involved really be explained?

One indication for an elective caesarean described by doctors constitutes a new phenomenon: tokophobia, which means a fear of contractions. One male midwife, Denis Walsh, has said he considers this fear to be socially created and he suggests it is a kind of iatrogenic fear (i.e. a fear caused by medicine or doctors), made stronger by the media, which generally supports the idea of medicalised birth (Walsh, 2002). Tokophobia is also caused by hearing about the bad experiences of friends and family, by impersonal treatment or by a lack of continuity of care.

Another writer, Dodwell, suggests that every woman who wants a caesarean should be able to talk to a midwife about this and look at alternative birthing possibilities, and then make an informed choice (Dodwell, 2002).

What does it mean to 'choose'?

It is necessary to have information when making a choice, but this alone is not sufficient. Choosing something is not an action but a process, which takes time, because it involves various stages. Within the technological model of birth making choices has become an obligation, which is fulfilled with the help of various numbers, abstract statistics and abstract information about potential risks.

You should be careful how you make decisions about the care you receive, or are to receive for birth... Take into account when knowledge is conveyed to you objectively, or whether you are steered towards making certain decisions. And consider how you feel about choice: are you happy to make choices, or would you prefer to be led towards an 'appropriate' choice? Much is said about freedom of choice and woman's so-called self-determination, but your unborn baby also needs to be taken into account. It has no choice... or does it? Perhaps its fate is already determined, i.e. its fate as regards the type of birth it needs for this life? Only you yourself can sense this. Listening to the baby within you, talking to him or her, helping him or her to become orientated towards the world... these are all important parts of the decision-making process. Make your choices about the care you receive or the actions you take while you are in contact with your baby, even early on in your pregnancy.

Also remember that the 'doctor' is no longer the person who dispenses knowledge and advice; instead he presents you with a series of possible, uncertain, medical procedures, which you are required to choose from—at your own risk. The fear we've already discussed is 'cured' by suggestions to have various medical interventions, which you are allowed... in fact *required* ... to choose between.

Nowadays, you have options you need to choose between

By requiring that you make choices, the problem of the complete uncertainty of the technology used in the field of childbirth is passed on to you and the need for ongoing 'choices' will lead you further and further away from what your body and your feelings are telling you. This will probably make you feel less and less capable of making a real choice and more and more in need of advice from so-called experts (Illich, 2005). Any advice you receive can actually never be objective because it will always be influenced by personal thoughts and experiences, by the advisor's social background and by many other factors. In any case, the information provided (for decision-making) will only appeal to your rational mind. A deep conflict is likely to arise between this kind of 'choice' and your personal experiences. There is likely to be a conflict between your 'social instinct' (i.e. your need to belong to a group) and your biological instinct (survival of the species and self-actualisation). If you make decisions purely on a rational level, you will probably be left with feelings of guilt and inadequacy. It's important for you to be aware of this conflict... Remember too, that any choice you make will always be influenced by your deep-seated needs and the fight-or-flight adaptation system. If you tune in to your deep feelings while making choices, you will often become aware of this problem, which lies behind the question of choice.

A free, true choice is bipolar: information is connected to your own feelings and intuition, which will give you a new perspective on your situation. It will take time to integrate these different aspects of the decision-making process, which will involve the opportunity to explore experience and feelings, experiment with possibilities, find new tools and find out about the physical aspects of your situation. In other words, it will involve everything which should be included in a good antenatal course. Difficult decisions are not taken quickly unless of course they are intuitively determined by the fight-or-flight response. It doesn't therefore make any sense for you to discuss your choice as regards caesarean section for half an hour in front of an anaesthetist... Give yourself time!

Choosing seems to be difficult because it means listening to yourself, coming to terms with your own ambivalence and working through it, taking responsibility and facing danger... as well as being attacked by other people or being shut out by them. *Not* choosing seems simple, because other people take over responsibility. The outcome is nevertheless precisely the other way round—*choosing* results in outcomes which are easier to deal with and *not choosing* results in outcomes which are very difficult to cope with. If you choose for herself, you will experience fulfilment, understanding, learning and growth. If you refuse to choose (and give up responsibility for your pregnancy, labour and birth) you will experience frustration, lack of understanding, conflict and a sense of alienation from your own self.

Making a choice results in outcomes which are easier to deal with. Not making a choice results in outcomes which are very difficult for you to cope with.

Photo © Sandro Pintus

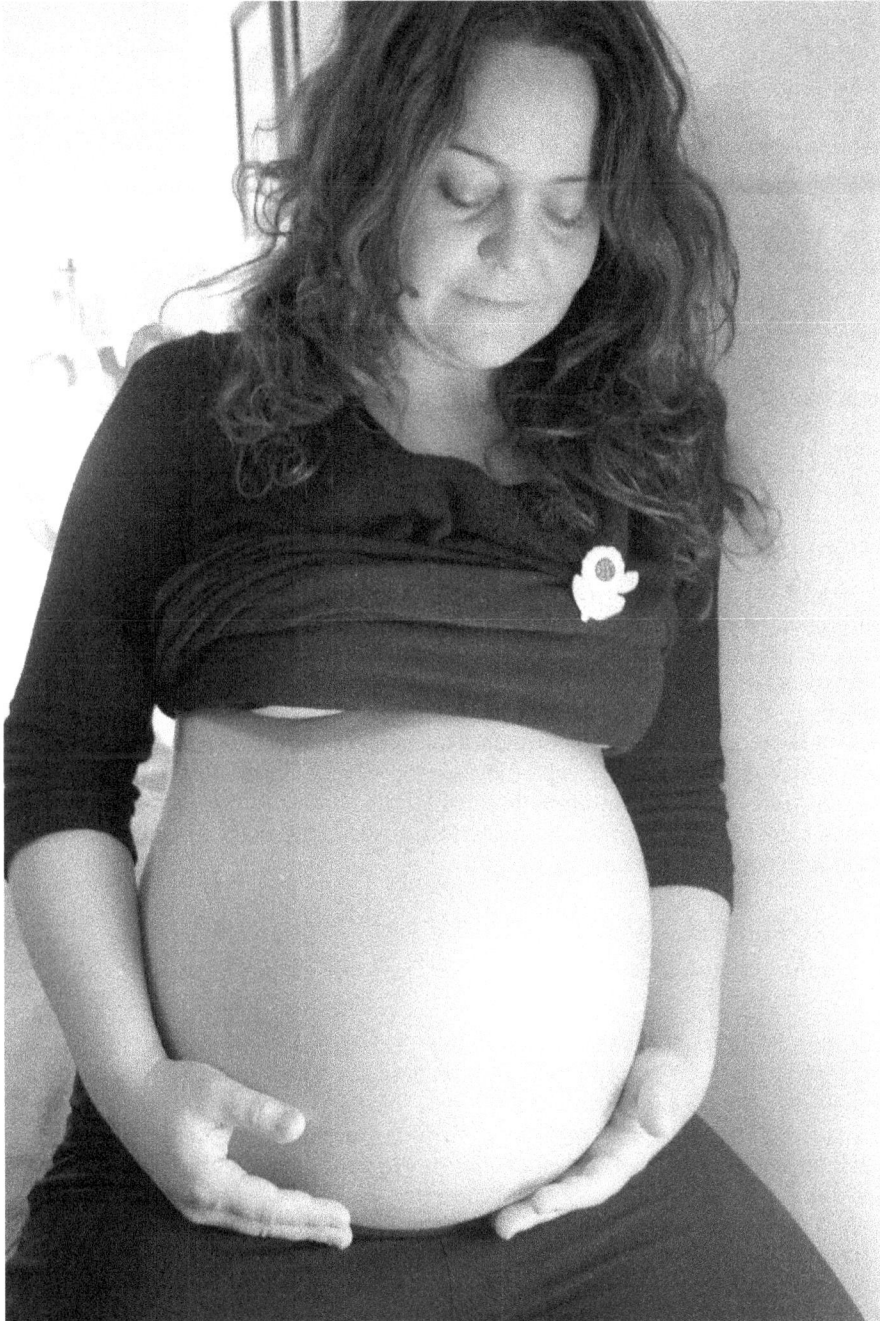

You need to integrate information, experience and intuition when making decisions

Finding support if you really want to have a caesarean

Although many consultants feel happy when women request a caesarean, midwives don't usually feel as comfortable. Often they feel distance ("She's having consultant-led care so what have I got to do with her?"), prejudice, frustration and anger ("She's second-guessing the birth—the part of all this which is so important for me," "She's not giving herself credit," "She's being selfish and just wants to be able to determine the date of the birth," etc). Midwives may also often feel a sense of failure, helplessness, disinterest and also a lack of empathy. Therefore, it's possible that you may not initially get a positive response if you request a caesarean from your usual midwife...

Or you may get an enthusiastic response, on the other hand. Even midwives have chosen a model of birth. If they have opted for the technological model, they may see the decision to have an elective caesarean as being just a surgical intervention without any further meaning. If, however, they have opted for the 'midwifery model' of birth, they would not then be ethically in agreement, but they would nevertheless not have any opportunity to approach you and so they would simply feel frustrated.

What feelings would you provoke in midwives?

I believe that many midwives have chosen the profession because they have been hurt or scarred during their own experiences of childbirth or in some other way which relates to their status as a woman. While midwives attend births, they experience the emotions of birth repeatedly and this allows them to heal themselves. But in order for this healing to take place they need experiences which symbolise success This means success for the women who we attend— while they are giving birth, while they are forming loving relationships with their babies and while they are breastfeeding. And if these positive experiences take place they confirm their ability to restore to wholeness to the 'dismembered woman' inside themselves.

When the processes of birth proceed smoothly, they confirm in midwives their ability to restore wholeness...

In reality, though, many of the women midwives attend are also injured. As a result, there are many difficult situations and difficult births. Perhaps midwives can nevertheless attend these births with empathy, but they are exhausting because the midwives have no sense of personal success. A woman in their care who misses out on this experience of wholeness, who denies her creative potential... this kind of woman is a real challenge for a midwife. Perhaps in these cases it is the midwife who should remind herself of the archetype of the 'dismembered woman' and in doing this find her way back to a sense of empathy. Through the awareness that women are all essentially *dismembered*, by remembering that women all have a centre of wholeness, midwives can potentially restore the situation to one of healing. After all, even a woman who is having an elective caesarean is transforming herself into a mother. And in order to do this, she just needs a little more help than other women. So even if you choose a caesarean, a midwife may be able to help you.

Photo © Sandro Pintus

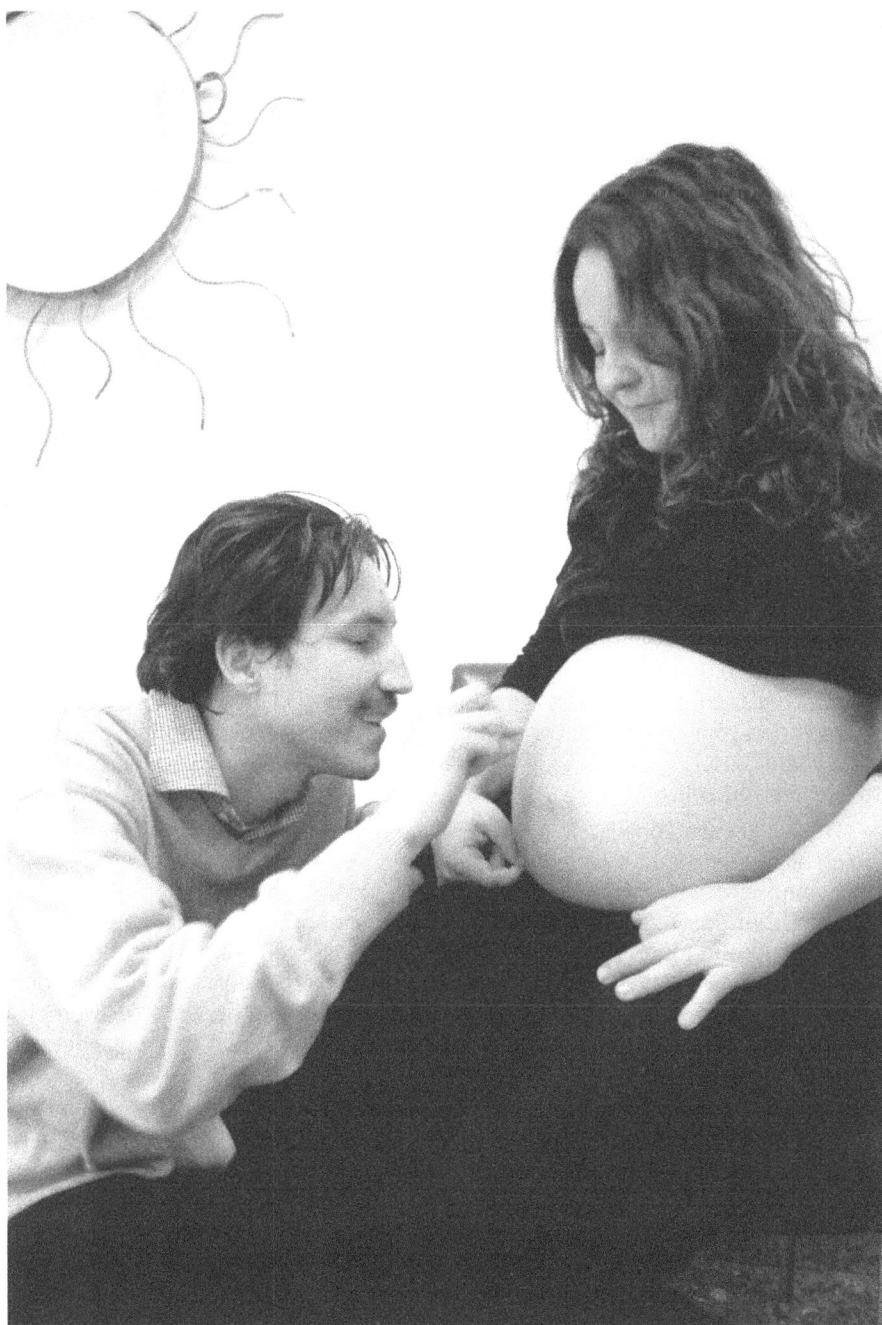

There are many difficult situations, and many difficult births as a result

Antenatal support if you are having an elective caesarean

If you choose to have an elective caesarean it is much less likely that you will seek out midwifery support or register for antenatal classes. The decision to have a caesarean is usually one which is taken with a consultant. However, in case you do seek out support from a midwife or doula, or even a friend, here are a few guidelines for getting maximum support from another person.

Since your choice (to have a caesarean) was probably made out of fear, because you must have an instinct to escape the act of giving birth or because you feel paralysed by the idea of it (having no 'weapons' to defend yourself from this threat), make sure you find a person who doesn't make you feel even more fearful and uncomfortable. (If the first person you talk to about your feelings is very negative and unhelpful, keep looking! You will eventually find someone who will be really supportive.) Look for a person who will listen to you and try to understand where your fear comes from. Then you can try to find ways of working towards a feeling of safety, with this person's support. And while you do this, focus on your feelings about your body and your growing baby.

If you want a caesarean, find someone who will listen to you and understand where your fear is coming from

Taking your fundamental needs as a starting point, your confidante can then try to offer you some new answers, which are different from those offered by medical technology. These can include giving you a sense of safety for yourself and your growing baby, helping you develop a feeling of 'integrity' and a feeling of connectedness with your baby and, finally, giving you the freedom to express yourself.

Talking to someone in this way will help you fulfil your personal needs, which all relate to your biological instincts. Also note that physical exercises will be helpful when you work with someone in this way, in an attempt to work through your feelings. This is because physical exercises will help you to become more in touch with your feelings. They will help you to breathe, relax, and have positive visualisations. Finally, physical exercises will strengthen your pelvic floor. Even sing, speak and exchange ideas with a group of other women, not just one. (See Chapters 5 and 6 for more information on relevant physical exercises.)

The information which you need to obtain if you are thinking about having a caesarean is that which relates to physiology and also that which will help you to perceive a connection between your bodily processes, your behaviour and your emotions. Your goal should be to tap into your own resources and work towards 'opening up', even if progress can only be made in tiny increments at a time. By working in this way, you will be able to feel more secure in yourself and you should even begin to understand the possibility of giving in to the process of childbirth.

It is particularly important to work in this way if you have requested an elective caesarean after the experience of rape or sexual abuse. And even if you have already had a previous caesarean section, this work will be meaningful. It is a matter of developing your ideas relating to protection (or defence), intimacy, support and the ability to say 'no', sharing, and acceptance.

Every woman's needs are related to her social instinct so it's useful if your feelings can be explored in a group setting. When doing any group work, it's vital that you share the group's values and develop a feeling of belonging to the group and also that your own personal values and ideas are validated. Make sure the group you join allows you to express and exchange ideas and feelings. Helpful topics for working on your needs during pregnancy and also during the birth (whatever kind of birth later takes place) include the following:

- **Support during pregnancy** It is vital that you receive support from people around you while you are pregnant, e.g. from your family and from your colleagues.
- **The setting for the birth itself** This should be a familiar place, where you feel safe, secure and protected... but which also feels intimate to you.
- **Birth attendants** You need to choose who your birth attendants are going to be. Anyone who is around you during the birth (particularly if you choose to go into labour and have your baby naturally) should not be anxious in any way or should at least be aware of his or her fears.
- **Help** Offers of help need to be realistic (instead of idealistic) so that you can develop realistic (not idealistic) expectations for the birth itself.

Since your social needs must be met, it's important that you find out about any procedures which are usually routine in the place where you're planning to go, that you know about different models of birth, about the historical development of midwifery and obstetrics, about strategies for dealing with suggested interventions, about choices you will have and also about ways in which you will be able to get support when you make decisions.

Your goal should be to minimise the possibility of any conflict between your biological and your social instincts—so that your stress levels are minimised. This work is particularly important if you are afraid of birth because of previously experienced iatrogenic (doctor-induced) problems. It is a question of discussing behaviour, decision-making and practising assertiveness, i.e. behaviour which relates to 'fighting.' In other words, you will be developing your survival instincts, which are valuable for ensuring a safe birth. In order to do this, you need to do the following:

- Make sure your fears are really 'heard' and listen to other women's fears too. This means you need to go beyond talking about risks and instead think about your personal situation. When your fear has a name and there is a concrete danger or problem, 'weapons' you can then develop 'weapons' in order to deal with this fear. For this to happen successfully, it's important that you explore all details of the concrete problem honestly, for example even talking about pain after a planned caesarean.

- Make an effort to respond more on an emotional level, so that you can more easily adapt to situations. Physical movements (exercises) and/or deep relaxation will help you to ease yourself out of any sense of numbness or paralysis and instead ease yourself into a natural rhythm. This process can take place during your pregnancy or after the birth. Alongside analytical thought, the instinctual ability to react will allow you to make informed choices, which respect your deep need for self-preservation and which preserve your integrity.
- Try to become increasingly aware of your growing baby's ability to respond because this is the foundation of its health, safety and life energy.

Become more aware of your baby's ability to respond

In order to achieve all of the above, you will need information about the healthy physiological processes of birth. Over time, you should develop a strong motivation to retain your instinct for self-preservation and your life energy. This work is particularly important if you are paralysed by fear. Continue working with other women after the birth too because all these approaches can be used either before or afterwards, i.e. they will help you heal long-term.

Support during the birth, if you're having an elective caesarean

Very often midwives meet women who want to have a caesarean for the very first time just before, during or after the intervention. What can be done about this? What do you think you'll need from your birth attendants if you're having a cesarean section?

Let's consider how you can choose a birth attendant for a caesarean…

- Find someone who seems to listen to you completely unjudgementally, who really seems to want to tune into your real needs. Perhaps you will find someone who will understand the specific fears and vulnerabilities which brought you to the point of preferring a caesarean section. If so, this birth attendant will be more likely to see you as a person, not as 'someone to watch' or 'a case', and this may alter the support you are offered.
- Find someone who will be a kind of 'psychological parent' for the experience of the birth (even if this continues to take place by caesarean section), for the process by which you bring your baby into the world and you become a mother. At the same time, find someone who will help you to come closer to understanding the rhythm and phases of becoming a mother, not someone who will only focus on the moment of the birth.

Find someone who will help you understand the rhythm and phases of becoming a mother, not just the birth

- Find someone who will be at your side when you get wheeled into theatre, who will tell you about the process of your baby's birth, who will help you to breathe through it, be with your baby, talk to him or her, help him or her adjust to being in the outside world and welcome him or her properly. If someone does these things, it will help you to start bonding with your baby, even if he or she has been born under difficult circumstances.
- Find someone who will stay close to you in the first few hours and days after the birth, because you will need help and support, you will be in pain and also you will have no hormonal underpinning for bonding and initial breastfeeding.
- If you have any difficulty relating to your new baby, find someone who will help you bring the father into the picture too. Encourage your birth attendant to explain to him the importance of properly orientating and welcoming the baby into this world. Should the father also not be in a position to do this, encourage your birth attendant to do this for you.
- Find someone who will help you to be as active as possible. Yes, you can be an active mother when an elective caesarean takes place! If you are active, it will help you to integrate part of yourself or at the very least to use some of the burst of energy which typically arises in the third trimester. Your baby comes into the world and perinatal psychology research suggests its personality is formed for its whole life. It needs help becoming orientated, it needs direction and support so as to be able to successfully separate from you and survive in the outside world. Your partner will become a father, his responsibilities will increase and he will need more strength so that he can become a good support within your family—so find a birth attendant who will support you in realising these goals. Encourage your birth attendant to help him grow into this new role and understand it properly.

Support after the birth, if you're having an elective caesarean

Just after the birth and in the months that follow the opening process continues even further. Your baby needs space near his or her parents, and you need to create this space. This process is more difficult when no natural physiological opening has taken place at the time of the birth. However, try to build up your physical strength through postnatal support and also in special postnatal classes, whose main aim is to promote and strengthen the mother-baby bond. If you are looking for a class, note the following are important:

- **Deep physical massage for your baby with some rhythmic pressure on his or her head** This will give your baby the uterine massage he or she missed during birth. In other words, it will imitate the natural processes of birth for your baby.
- **Exercises to stimulate your baby** These will help your baby to respond, make instinctive decisions and fight for survival. Exercises can include, for example, daily baby baths and massages, 'baby gymnastics'—sometimes classes are available!—as well as making signs to your baby, recognising his or her attempts at communication, responding appropriately and providing other forms of mental stimulation.

- **Practising the rhythm of symbiosis and separation** This can involve putting your baby under water at a swimming pool, then bringing him or her to the surface again, pushing him or her away, then pulling him close again, or passing your baby back and forth between you and your partner.
- **Exercises which help** you **trust** your **baby** These constitute a form of 're-bonding. One method is for you to be massaged while you are lying in bed, in an intimate atmosphere, and for your baby to be bathed next to you, also in a relaxed, calm and intimate way. After the bath, your wet baby is then put on your naked breasts, you are both covered and left alone. These conditions, which are similar to those which often occur after a natural birth, will stimulate you to produce hormones (oxytocin and prolactin) and they will help you to bond and breastfeed successfully.

Being able to 'separate' is closely connected with trust and letting go. You and your baby will be constantly confronted with the need to separate in your lives. In a caesarean birth, the process of separation is incomplete. If you and your baby are unable to experience this separation at the time of the birth, it can be consciously practised afterwards. Your partner can play an important role in this by taking care of your baby. Not only will that help to reduce your stress levels, it will also help you to bond with your baby and breastfeeding is then also more likely to develop smoothly.

Often, a few months after giving birth, women experience feelings of guilt or failure

Debriefing birth experiences is also important because often—after a few months—feelings of guilt or failure come to the surface. It is important to understand which feelings are caused by external factors and which ones come from you yourself. When you understand this you will be able to dismiss external causes (to a certain extent) and learn from those factors which relate to you. This will help you to restore your sense of trust and help you to learn from what you've recently experienced. If you relearn how to trust yourself this will also help your child to learn how it can trust itself.

In conclusion, I would like to emphasise that all this is to do with really exploring the real situation relating to you and your baby and the pain and feelings you experience. It's a question of being present to your own experiences and feelings and your baby's, and using the normal, natural processes as a focus and a means of healing, even though the times and rhythms of these have been forced out of synch through the intervention of the caesarean operation. It is possible to rebuild the natural processes in a certain sense and somehow promote and support the processes of renewal. Any birth partner's or friend's talk, as I see it, involves helping you accept and extend limits. In order for this to happen successfully, I suggest you see healing as a path to follow, not as a goal in itself.

See healing as a path to follow, not as a goal

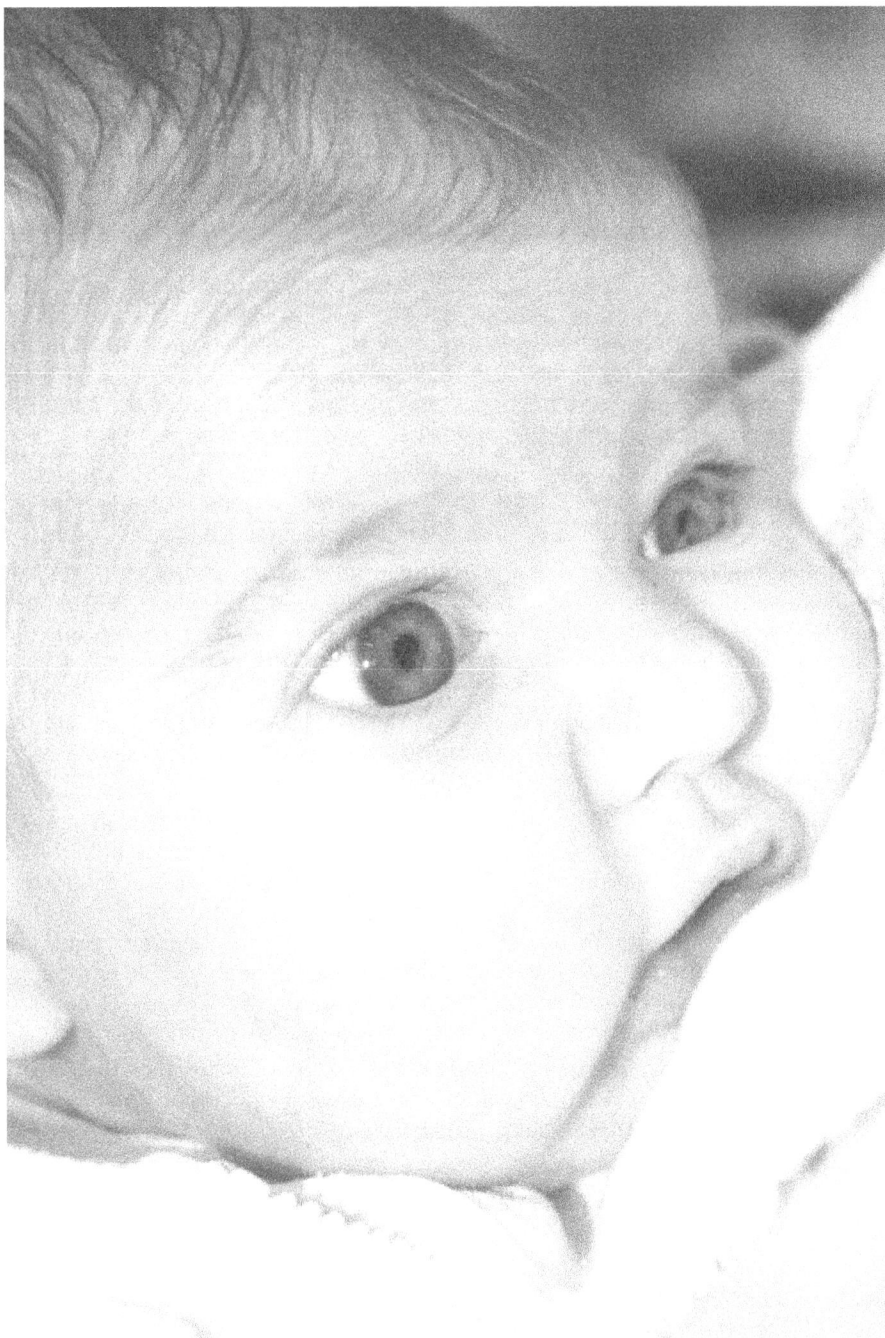

You need to consider your baby's experience too, whenever you make decisions

CHAPTER 4:

Drug-based pain relief

The purpose of pain relief and the risks associated with it

According to Prof G Pescetto, an obstetrician and gynaecologist who co-authored an Italian manual of obstetrics and gynaecology in the late 1960s, pain relief must be harmless for both mother and baby. It should remove pain or reduce it. It should not inhibit contractions nor interfere with the activity of the relevant muscles in the second stage of labour. Even after the birth, it should not prevent the contraction and retraction of the uterus.

Beyond these necessary conditions I would add that pain relief for you while you're in labour should always leave you in a state of full consciousness so that you are able to uninhibitively experience the joy of becoming a mother.

Unfortunately, no method of medical pain relief is completely risk-free for your baby and free of side-effects for you. Risks exist partly because of the technology used, partly because of the chemical effect of pharmaceuticals used, and partly because any intervention disturbs the normal physiological processes of labour and birth. Unwanted side-effects can reveal themselves straight after pain relief is administered or much later, and can have a short- or long-term impact. These side-effects may be very obvious or they may be very difficult to detect.

Every drug-based method of pain relief reaches the fetus within a few seconds of being administered. Even when any damaging effects of pain relief cannot be proven afterwards, the possibility that they exist cannot be dismissed. And not all damage can be established directly after the birth using the very crude assessments which are typically used (the Apgar score, blood analyses, etc). Slow-acting effects have hardly been researched. It has been possible to significantly reduce some risks by lowering the dosage of certain types of pain relief, but the risks have not been completely eliminated.

There are clear correlations between medical pain relief and long-term damage to the central nervous system. The following have been observed in newborns whose mothers used drug-based pain relief (Buckley, 2005; Leighton, *et al*, 2002):

- later or altered sensory and motor reactions
- a reduced ability to process afferent stimuli
- a reduced ability to react appropriately to afferent stimuli
- disturbances with rooting and sucking reflexes (and consequently babies' ability to obtain nourishment) and even the crawling reflex
- irritability and excitability
- reduced tolerance of stress

- respiratory depression
- altered muscle tone
- increased incidence of newborn jaundice
- bluish colouring of the skin
- disturbed sleep rhythms
- jitteriness

The more pain relief the labouring woman received, the more frequently these effects were observed. What's more, the effect of drug-based pain relief on the course of labour and birth almost always constitutes dystocia—i.e. a slowing down of the natural, physiological processes—which results in the need for IV-administered augmentation. The labouring woman loses control and can no longer continue to work consciously with her contractions. Nevertheless, pain is often only slightly reduced. The first contact between the mother and newborn after the birth is often disturbed, since both parties are still tired and dazed or drugged. Relationship problems and difficulties with breastfeeding are often the result.

Epidural and spinal anaesthesia

This seems to be the most frequently used and also the most effective method of pain relief but it is also the most invasive. Of these two forms of anaesthesia, epidurals are administered in either problematic or normal labours, while spinals are only used for caesarean sections. For both forms of anaesthesia, it is a question of administering an anaesthetic drug mixed with opiates (which are partly narcotic). In the case of a normal labour or long labours epidural anaesthesia is used in lower doses. In both cases, the drugs (e.g. bupivacaine, ropivacaine, fentanyl and sufentanil) are injected into the epidural space (at the 3rd or 4th lumbar vertebrae) by means of a catheter. The drugs are either continuously injected or administered according to the woman's request, or self-administered.

Insufficient research has been carried out into epidurals and spinals. Even if the safety of the technology has been proven, controlled studies following mothers who've had epidurals have not looked at long-term effects on both mothers and babies and they have not considered sufficiently high numbers of cases. Many studies focus only on how drugs can be combined and on the dose possibilities of the drugs injected.

EFFECTIVENESS

Epidurals are often considered to be the most effective form of pain relief and this has been corroborated by studies, particularly when opiates are used in the epidural mix (MIDIRS, 1997). As well as generally evaluating the pain relief as 'very good', many women who've had an epidural once are happy to have one a second time. Only a small number of women rate epidurals as being 'not very effective'.

TECHNICAL DIFFICULTIES

An incorrectly administered epidural may occasionally lead to partial or full paralysis or long-term disturbances to nerve sensitivity (e.g. paraesthesia)—and it may be only partially effective as pain relief. In addition, there is the possibility of neurological complications, infections, epidural or subarachnoid haemorrhage, loss of spinal fluid (which results in bad migraines), and hypotonia.

Epidurals imply various risks and side-effects

SIDE-EFFECTS AND EFFECTS ON THE DYNAMICS AND PROCESS OF BIRTH

- The need for the use of intravenous oxytocics (i.e. syntocinon—artificial oxytocin) is often reported as being significantly higher in epidural births than in normal births (Mayberry, 2002). When women do not perceive any pain, paradoxically they also do not experience the stimulus to produce oxytocin, so their contractions become weaker and less regular. Uterine activity is reduced. And although it is possible to reactivate uterine activity using synthetic oxytocin, it is not possible to have any influence over the delayed opening up of the cervix.
- As a result of decreased muscle tone in the uterus, there seems to be a higher incidence of malpresentation or abnormal fetal lie. In addition, the first stage of labour becomes longer (in normal labour) and this involves risks for both mother and baby—as has already been mentioned.
- The use of ventouse, forceps and episiotomy is three times as common as in normal births (Buckley, 2005).
- When epidural dosage is well controlled and when the dose is decreased during the second stage of labour, although there are fewer instrumental deliveries many women find the pain unbearable. This is because they have not gradually been able to get used to it and because no endorphins have been produced. No doubt, this pain is much worse than that which women would have experienced in a natural, undrugged birth (Buckley, 2005).
- If a fully-dilated woman receives directions on how to push (commanded or directed pushing), without actually feeling the impulse to push (which is often the case in epidural births), forceps are often applied so as to support rotation of the unborn baby's head. According to research, delaying pushing efforts for 90 minutes results in significant decreases in the amount of time women spent pushing (Kelly, *et al,* 2010).
- A woman's ability to move around is often inhibited and this can result in the loss of other physical perception. Not feeling any need to urinate, for example, can necessitate the use of a urinary catheter.
- Hypotension in the woman can cause fetal bradycardia (a slowing of the heartbeat). An increase in maternal temperature (as a result of the epidural) may also often result in fetal tachycardia (the opposite).
- Life-threatening complications occur in a small number of cases. Maternal death caused by the use of an epidural is extremely rare but not unknown.

- Epidurals have no obvious effect on newborn Apgar scores or on the pH values of fetal blood. Detailed neurological research has revealed negative effects on muscle tone and on newborn behaviour. The lower the dose of drugs used, the less these effects are recorded (Buckley, 2005; Leighton, 2002). In one randomised controlled study on children's behaviour five years after their birth, no differences could be found between children born with an epidural and those born without one (Leighton, 2002).
- After experiencing an epidural the mother can have a mild or even a bad headache lasting up to 10 days. In some cases these headaches can last up to six weeks (Leighton, 2002).
- Serious neurological damage in the woman is extremely rare but not unheard of. A small number of women report feeling weak for around three months postnatally and experience loss of sensation.
- Although this has not yet been sufficiently researched, there are reports and clinical observations of long-term pain in the lumbar vertebrae and in the area of the sacrum.
- In the case of 'mobile' epidurals, the dosage of local anaesthetic (e.g. bupivacaine) is very weak and it is mixed with an opiate (such as fentanyl), both of which are injected via a catheter. The woman retains her ability to move around, and her ability to feel herself moving is not dramatically impaired. One randomised controlled trial, which compared the 'conventional epidural' (i.e. the non-mobile one) with the lower-dose one, which mixed in opiates, was not able to establish any difference in birth mode (i.e. whether the women ended up giving birth vaginally, or needing a caesarean, forceps or ventouse). However, there was a high rate of lower blood pressure, headaches and pruritis (itching) in the 'mobile' group (MIDIRS, 1997). Women preferred this method, but more research needs to be carried out into unwanted side-effects, particularly with respect to the use of opiates.

GENERAL SIDE-EFFECTS OF LOCAL ANAESTHETICS

- On the labouring woman side-effects include: atony of the myometrium, reduced muscle tone, a lowering of blood pressure, tachycardia (palpitations), dizziness, nausea and breathlessness.
- On the fetus side-effects include: bradycardia (or reactive tachycardia), high levels of acidosis at birth (increased acid in the blood), a depressive effect on the heart muscles, changes in the development of muscles, eyesight and nerves.
- In both mother and baby the use of local anaesthetic can have damaging effects on the central nervous system. Of course, the frequency and severity of these side-effects depend on how high and for how long a dose of narcotics was used. It is nevertheless incorrect to maintain that these side-effects do not occur with low doses. The local anaesthetic passes across the placental barrier and is therefore always absorbed by the fetus. Side-effects are rare, but not completely unheard of.

- Quite apart from the risks already known (which we have already listed) the opiates used may have another long-term effect on the baby. During the critical phase of puberty, adolescents whose mothers received opiates during labour have a higher susceptibility to drug addiction (Jacobsen, 1988; Jacobsen, 1990). Jacobsen suggested that this is because of a mechanism to do with oxytocin that fixes the memories of birth and biochemical feedback in the involuntary part of the mind, whereby adolescents react to oxytocin production in puberty, so that these memories are reactivated (Jacobsen, 1988; Jacobsen, 1990). Until now there has been no research to determine whether or not this phenomenon also occurs when opiates are used in epidurals. What we do know, though, for sure, is that these opiates cross the placenta and enter the fetus.

Local anaesthetics can have damaging effects

KEY POINTS ABOUT EPIDURALS

Since epidurals are the most effective method of pain relief, they are very popular with women. However, since epidurals also represent the most invasive method and result in the highest number of complications, it is important that you are able to make an *informed choice*, before you go into labour or at least that you can do so when contractions begin. The information you receive must be comprehensive and honest and both the pros and cons of epidurals must be detailed. In any case, note the following...

- You need to find out whether or not epidurals are available every day and during the night and also how long it takes for the pain relief to take effect from the time a decision is made to have an epidural. When you request an epidural either the infrastructure or the anaesthetists are not always available for the epidural to be arranged immediately. While you are waiting you are then no longer motivated to actively deal with your labour pain, because you will have set your mind on having an epidural. Therefore, you also need to be fully informed about alternative possibilities. You should also be informed of the availability of mobile epidural anaesthesia, and of the extent to which mobility might be possible.
- Anaesthesia cannot be used in early labour. Also, take into account the fact that many practitioners prefer anaesthesia to wear off by the beginning of the second stage so that you can at least tackle part of the work of birth with your own strength. Whether you have an epidural or not you will almost certainly be expected to get through the birth itself without the help of your body's natural compensatory mechanisms (which would no longer be working smoothly, because of the disturbance the anaesthesia causes).
- In order to reduce epidural side-effects to a minimum and avoid disturbances to the physiological mechanisms of birth as far as possible, it is best if you request an epidural as late as possible and if the lowest possible dose of anaesthesia is used. The aim of your caregivers is to reduce your perception of pain while not completely shutting it out.

Epidurals are the most invasive method of pain control

- As a result of using epidurals, the costs of healthcare increase. On the one hand this is because of the intervention itself and on the other it is because of the consequent increase in instrumental or operative deliveries and later health problems. This will probably only interest you if you are paying for your care within a private system of health!

- The higher the epidural rate, the higher the rate of associated problems. A group of resident doctors here in England, where approximately 25% of women labour with an epidural, have embarked on a government research project which is looking into the already well-known side-effects of epidurals. They claim they have observed an increase in the number of spinal complications with incurable consequences and disabilities. One of these doctors, Roger Godsiff, believes that the kind of epidural that is used to ease the pain of birth triggers a vicious circle of damage to the central nervous system.

- As far as I know, there has as yet been no research to compare medical attempts at pain relief with natural methods, comparing them in terms of side-effects, the labour process, maternal satisfaction, postnatal depression and effects on the newborn baby.

- It also hasn't yet been considered how far epidurals determine the nature of the birthing experience for you and your baby. Knowing what we know about the physiology of birth, we can say that if you have your pain taken away from you while you're in labour you will also be deprived of all other forms of emotional stimulation and compensatory mechanisms. As a result, you would be robbed of an experience of self discovery and also of the intense fulfilment which comes from achieving something through your own effort. The only thing that (probably) remains unaffected is your love for your baby. Having said that, though, we do know now that the hormonal cocktail of birth hormones is important not only for pain relief, but also for the protection and bonding process with your baby. Animals don't accept their offspring without these hormones and although human beings have affective and cultural tools to start a relationship with a new baby, on a deep biological level the bonding process is surely disturbed and your baby would miss out on natural imprinting processes.

- Natural methods of pain relief (which I will be talking about in the next chapter) may offer a similar level of relief from pain, without the risks which accompany the use of epidurals.

WHEN IS AN EPIDURAL RECOMMENDED?

Compared to all the risks and side-effects of an epidural, a labour which is proceeding naturally is far, far healthier and offers all kinds of advantages. Therefore, the use of an epidural can only be justified when it is medically indicated and if you are making a fully informed choice.

It is different in the case of dystocia (failure to progress), in which case an epidural can serve an important therapeutic function. If you are very fearful and tense when you're in labour, which would mean you wouldn't be able to relax during the breaks between your contractions, stress and adrenaline levels would remain high. Endorphin production would be inhibited and your sympathetic nervous system would become overstimulated. This would increase the level of pain you would experience in an unnatural way, meaning that your cervix and the lower segment of your uterus would become rigid, uterine contractions would go into spasm, there would be reduced flow of blood through the placenta and, finally, there would even be a danger that your unborn baby might suffer from hypoxia (lack of oxygen). In this kind of case an epidural would dissolve your stress and fear and make it possible for you to relax your muscle tone and cervix, and therefore the situation would also improves for your unborn baby. Only in this situation is it possible to see fast progress towards birth when an epidural is inserted and it is only in this case that the advantages of epidurals outweigh their possible side-effects. After all, very often the stress a labouring woman experiences is caused by the hospital environment itself, or by a lack of sensitive, loving support. An economical and effective approach would be for healthcare systems to invest in midwifery services. With suitable training, and given sufficient time and space—one-to-one care—midwives can help you a great deal in labour by reducing your stress levels and bringing your pain down to its physiological minimum.

If ever an epidural seems a good idea while you're in labour, focus on staying in good contact with your unborn baby. With an epidural in place your baby might suddenly feel alone (since you would no longer be groaning or moving around, or sending him or her supporting hormones). It is therefore good if you can communicate to your baby that it is *not* alone and that its further help is important. If you consciously breathe 'towards' your unborn child, this feeling of separation can be overcome, and at the same time your conscious breathing will help you to feel relaxed and in control. While this is happening, your partner (the baby's father) can also play an important role if he lays his hands on the your bump and talks to the baby you have made together.

Often a woman experiences stress in hospital

Sedatives and narcotic analgesia

In using drug-based pain relief, an attempt is made to control pain on two levels. Firstly, there is an attempt to manage pain on the afferent pain pathways and secondly, there is an attempt to manage it in the structures of your central nervous system. In order to block pain in the afferent pain pathways, it is necessary to use local anaesthesia, which blocks your nerve trunk. (This is the case with the pudendal block and the paracervical block, neither of which are used much nowadays—although they are considered very useful in poor resource countries.) In order to effect pain control through your central nervous system, sedatives or narcotic analgesia need to be used.

SEDATIVES

These have a sedative (calming) effect in relation to your fear and worry and would promote a sense of emotional well-being, rest and sleep. In addition, sedatives reduce nausea and vomiting. They work on the affective-motivational dimension of pain and would have a calming and inhibiting effect on your baby and on its life-sustaining functions.

- Fast-acting barbiturates, such as Seconal and Nembutol are often used in some countries, even today, because of their immediately calming effect. (However, they are rarely used in the UK.) They are used in some places even though this type of barbiturate can be detected in both the mother's and baby's body for a long time after the birth, and even though they may make the mother-to-be feel 'oppressed' and cause fetal repiratory depression.

- Tranquilisers such as Diazepam (e.g. Valium®) are still widely used. These inhibit memory and reduce maternal fear and worry. They weaken the barrier created by local anaesthetics, making them less effective. They would also lower your unborn baby's blood pressure and would be detected in your newborn baby 36-48 hours after the birth. Your baby's heart rate would flatten (i.e. it would show no signs of change) and, postnatally, your baby might suffer from respiratory depression, oedema (swelling), abnormal reflexes and, consequently, he or she might also have problems feeding and swallowing (i.e. when breastfeeding or formula feeding). It is likely that you would experience nausea and drowsiness, that you would lose conscious control and that you would fall into a state of hypotonia. You might also develop paradoxical reactions, such as restlessness and excitability. In addition, this drug may cause respiratory depression in the you during labour, which consequently causes hypoxia (lack of oxygen) in your unborn baby (Bonica, 1977).

NARCOTIC ANALGESIA

Mostly, morphine derivatives are used (like pethidine or diamorphine). The idea is that morphine stimulates the nerves of your brain stem and thereby has an inhibitive effect on the information in your body (in the sensory-perceptive dimension) and on the activity in your neocortex (in the cognitive-evaluating dimension). Narcotics are used during the active stage of labour but never in the second stage. Sometimes they are used in combination with sedatives in a 'cocktail'. The pain-inhibiting effect is not very strong, but during labour you would no longer be in a position to react to pain and express it.

Pethidine has numerous side-effects including nausea, dizziness, limited consciousness, and breathlessness in the breaks between contractions. Your unborn baby would also be likely to suffer from respiratory depression, have difficulties sucking and swallowing and have problems adapting to life outside your womb. These effects can last for days or, in some cases, even weeks.

Sedatives and narcotics inhibit many natural bodily processes, such as the natural production of endorphins (with well-known consequences). This causes difficulties during the first phase of your relationship with your baby (involving bonding and breastfeeding). Nevertheless, the main characteristic of this form of pain relief is that it would make you passive. In other words, you would *suffer* labour and birth instead of actively experiencing it and actively shaping its development. Your baby would also begin his or her life numbed and drugged, and incapable of reacting and adapting to his or her new environment.

With pethidine, etc the baby begins his or life numbed

Inhalation analgesia (Entonox / gas and air)

Inhalation analgesia, which uses a 50/50 mixture of nitrous oxide and oxygen, is often used in Britain and Scandinavia, as well as in other former British colonies (such as India), but it is rarely used in other countries in Europe or in the USA. In Britain, it is even used in home births. The advantage of this form of pain relief is that you can regulate the dosage yourself and also you only need to inhale the drug during contractions (not continuously), when you feel you need it. Only small quantities of the gas would be stored in your body and the drug would be quickly removed from both your own and your baby's body.

Side-effects of this form of drug-based pain relief depend on the dosage used and on the length of time you inhale the gas. Inhalation analgesia could result in respiratory depression (i.e. problems breathing) and depression of the central nervous system for both you and your baby. It could also be damaging to your kidneys, to a certain extent.

Even with this narcotic method of pain relief, it would be essential for a midwife to be present when you used it, so that your need for the gas could be minimised.

Conclusions and challenges for you and your midwives

If the complex and individualistic mechanisms of labour pain are taken into account, it is clear that all the medical forms of pain relief we have discussed are only partially effective. They fulfil only part of the requirements of an 'ideal' form of pain relief, while the rest remain unmet. When you are offered drug-based pain relief (with all its side-effects) there is a real contradiction... On the one hand you have been advised during the whole of your pregnancy to avoid drugs in all situations, because they might be harmful to your baby. On the other, while you are in labour you are offered drugs which have countless damaging effects on both you and your baby. The main reason for this contradiction is that there is neither the time, nor the staff to treat every 'case' as an individual person. This is unfortunate because pain can only be dealt with on an individual, holistic basis.

Through your whole pregnancy you have been told to avoid drugs, then you are offered them during labour

Clearly, it is important for you to decide for yourself what's important to you. After you have been given comprehensive information about possibilities and risks you can write a birth plan or 'care guide' (see Chapter 6). This might force you to think about drug-based pain relief as well as about the kind of support you want to have for the birth and the kind of environment you want to be in, in order to feel safe. Writing a birth plan (or care guide) might also help you to think through where you want to give birth to your baby and it might help you to think about what might be useful to you in that situation. Of course, you will also need to take any special needs of yours into account, whether these are emotional or physical in nature.

As early as 1962 a researcher called Buxton stated that interpersonal relationships and environment were inextricably linked (Buxton, 1962). He suggested that attending births professionally should be nothing more than an extension and refinement of the old practice of providing loving attention with boundless understanding, which has always been the most important aspect of providing birthing support, whoever provides it and wherever the people happen to be. Buxton finished by saying that this 'attention' has been neglected for two reasons: firstly, because birth has been moved from the home into hospitals, and secondly, because patient amnesia has become the highest goal. The net result has been to make the experience of childbirth as impersonal as possible.

Daniel Friedman emphasised the differences between home and hospital environments in connection with birth stress (Friedmann, 1974). He suggested that a labouring woman's stress begins when she leaves the intimate, warm and cosy atmosphere of her home and steps into the cold, sterile atmosphere of the hospital. Lesser and Keane proposed that you have five basic needs when you are in labour (Lesser and Keane, 1956):

- You will need to have a trusted support person.
- You will need to have your pain acknowledged and you will need strategies to relieve and cope with that pain.
- You will need the reassurance that the outcome of the birth will be good for both you and your baby.
- You will need acceptance from your birth attendants, irrespective of how you behave or how you personally see birth.
- You will need to be taken care of physically.

Bonica described the dilemma which doctors face in relation to drug-based pain relief (Bonica, 1977). He suggested that attending labouring women who are not using any pain relief requires more investment of physical and emotional energy. If all a doctor's patients were given this attention (or if they wanted it?) this would constitute an intolerable situation for some male doctors and would also not be manageable for maternity staff catering for normal birth. He said this was an insoluble problem because doctors are not in a position to get involved with the rediscovered needs of labouring women.

Perhaps midwives can solve this problem? Perhaps you need to ask them!

CHAPTER 5:

Drug-free approaches to pain relief

Natural pain relief does not aim to completely obliterate your labour pain. Instead, it aims to reduce it to its physiological minimum. Beyond this, it aims to help you develop an accepting attitude. It also aims to ensure that the experience of birth remains a 'whole-person' experience for you .

Principles behind the idea of sensory control

Controlling pain during labour and birth can actually be achieved by increasing your normal level of physical activity. Sensory control is based on the idea of stimulating nerves which have an inhibitory effect on pain transmission. These nerves can be reached using physiological means and by working on the sensory-perceptive dimension. Free nerve endings are activated using light, superficial stimuli, while your corpuscular (specialised) nerve endings react to temperature, movement and deep pressure and are responsible for the stimuli which penetrate to a much deeper level.

It is important to appreciate the laws which govern how stimuli are transmitted

At this point, it is important to appreciate the laws which govern how these stimuli are transmitted. First, there is the law of slightest intensity, which is the minimum intensity needed to activate any transmission. Secondly, there is the law of minimal energy increase, which is the amount of increase that causes an appreciable increase in sensation. Finally, there is the law of adaptation, which means that you will no longer notice a stimulus of the same intensity after a certain period of time. This is the habituation effect (Bonica, 1977).

Tools for achieving sensory control

Sensory methods of control include TENS (transcutaneous electrical nerve stimulation), intracutaneous sterile water injections, massage, the use of hot or cold compresses, audio analgesia and to some extent also acupuncture.

TENS (TRANSCUTANEOUS ELECTRICAL NERVE STIMULATION)

This method selectively activates your large nerve fibres using weak electrical stimulation. This allows the pain barrier in the posterior horns of your spine to close, and the T-cells, which normally transmit painful stimuli to your brain, to become blocked. Weak electrical stimulation is conveyed over electrodes which are applied to your back and stuck to your skin. Using this method of electrical stimulation for 20-30 minutes could significantly reduce your pain for several hours.

This method has varying degrees of popularity even though machines have now improved markedly. Nowadays there are small TENS devices specially designed for use in labour. You can use these machines when you are on your own and they can be switched off during pauses between contractions. In this way you can decide when you want stimulation and how much stimulation you want.

RCTs could not find any significant reduction in pain

Several randomised controlled studies were not able to establish any significant reduction in pain in women using TENS, compared to women not using TENS (Van der Spank, 2000). Nevertheless, women themselves seem very ready to accept this technology because TENS makes them feel that they are directing and controlling the pain themselves.

If, at the same time as using TENS, the affective-motivational dimension of pain is activated, the success rate of this method increases significantly. TENS then becomes a good method for mediating the fear women have of natural birth, particularly in hospitals, before an epidural is decided upon.

INTRACUTANEOUS OR HYPERTONIC STERILE WATER INJECTIONS

In this technique 0.1ml of sterile water (hypotonic) is injected underneath your skin. The most effective points for injections are: one finger above the lumbo-sacral joint and three fingers below the first injection. Recent research has shown, that this method is more effective than acupuncture, but for some reason acupuncture is carried out more often.[50] Martensson *et al* show that with sterile water injections pain relief, relaxation and subjective acceptance of sensations is better than with acupuncture (although there is no difference between the two methods in terms of requests for further pain relief) (Martensson, *et al*, 2008). Intracutaneous sterile water injections can dissolve intense pain for a period of one to two hours. They are effective as pain relief because the injection gives a sharp but short pain—which activates your fast-moving pain pathways, stimulates your brain stem and activates its pain-reducing mechanism of endorphin production and gate control. The method therefore works on the sensory-perceptive dimension. With just one injection, pain relief can be achieved for a few hours.

MASSAGE AND TOUCH

These also work on the sensory-perceptive dimension using direct stimulation by applying pressure in different ways. Both massage and movement also work on the affective-motivational dimension thanks to the fact that they both involve loving touch. The style of massage should therefore show the masseur's empathy and engagement with you, as well as respecting the physiological laws of stimulus transfer. The following points should be taken into account when a birth partner uses massage on you:

- Applying counter-pressure on the parts of your body which are painful will activate underlying receptors and corpuscular nerve endings. For this reason it is best if you are massaged *during* contractions.
- Gentle, superficial movements will activate your skin receptors and free nerve endings. It is best, therefore, if this massage style is used during *breaks* between contractions.
- From time to time, the intensity of touch or the style of massage should be changed, so as to prevent you from getting used to a particular intensity or style (which would make the massage less effective). Your sensations while you're in labour are likely to be very clear, so you will usually be able to say what type and strength of contact you would like and where you would like to have it.

HOT AND COLD COMPRESSES

Compresses can be damp (in the case of wet packs and folded cloths) or dry (in the case of warm bottles, ice packs, bean bags or warmed salt in cloth). They should either be used alternately or in any way you feel you need them. They will have an effect on your nerve endings which is similar to that which occurs during massage. In addition, if compresses are applied to your back, they will help to reduce tension in your muscles and ligaments. The birth attendant or caregiver who uses compresses needs to be careful to avoid both hot and cold burns.

AUDIO ANALGESIA

By intense stimulation of your sense of hearing through headphones, it is possible to reduce your fear and your expectation of pain. You or your birth attendants can use various sounds, such as stereo music, neutral background noises (such as ocean waves or a gurgling brook) or 'white noise' (i.e. sounds of a constant volume, which are even in each frequency band, such as 'snow' on the television). Audio analgesia will activate a complex system which will allow your pain threshold to increase. A calming of your reticular system seems to occur.

ACUPUNCTURE

Acupuncture passes through the sensory-perceptive dimension and seems to affect your whole energy system, when it's used. This technique involves inserting thin needles into special points on 'meridians' (energy lines running round your body). The needles may then be moved around, turned or regularly stimulated with an electrical current (with breaks in between). We can hypothesise that this may allow central systems to be stimulated, so that inhibiting (pain-lowering) impulses are sent to your posterior horns or your afferent nerves, so that the production of endorphins is stimulated.

The pain-relieving effect will usually only occur after 15-20 minutes and it can last for several hours if direct stimulation continues. Pain relief will only be partial but pain certainly seems to be reduced in most women and they say it therefore becomes bearable. Above all, acupuncture might make it easier for you to achieve a deep state of relaxation during breaks between contractions—which would be a significant contribution to pain relief. This method of pain relief would minimise your tension and fear of pain and would not affect your state of mind. As a result, it should not negatively influence your experience of birth. However, it would affect your freedom of movement to some extent. Similar effects can be obtained through acupressure and this would allow you to move around more freely.

If you decide to use acupuncture or acupressure it is of course important that you make sure they are administered by a person who is fully trained in these forms of pain relief.

Principles behind the idea of psychological control

In order to use methods of psychological control, we need to gain a better understanding of the psychological mechanisms at work during pregnancy, labour and birth. This means we will also need to reconsider the nature of labour pain, the nature of any fears you may have and also the effect stress might have on your pregnancy and on your experience of labour and birth. Coming to a better understanding of all these elements of your experience will help us to understand why certain methods of psychological control have been proposed and also why they are reported to be effective.

THE NATURE OF LABOUR PAIN

If we focus on the central characteristics of pain, we encounter a complex, profound, *primal* world. After all, although we can name the various parts of the brain and order these into affective, instinctive and cognitive functions, pain seems to go way beyond this physiology and seems to affect people at the very core of their being.

If we remind ourselves that labour pain—contractions of uterine muscles and the pain this involves—along with love, is the first experience and 'imprinting' which a human being receives, then it is also easier to understand its fundamental purpose. This purpose is to communicate that life is a dynamic process which flows between two contrasting and mutually-defining poles of experience, i.e. *contraction* (which involves effort and strength or a feeling of malaise, pain and discomfort) and *expansion* (which involves feelings of well-being, relaxation and love). One 'pole' cannot exist without the other. Without this polarity, love itself would be inert and have no form of expression. Even breathing, the first life-giving function we experience, moves us between the poles of contraction and expansion. In fact, the first thing we do when we are born is breathe in... and the last thing we do is breathe out—we *expire*.

We need to understand that hardship and suffering belong to life in just the same way as joy and a sense of well-being. When we live within this rhythm we grow and continue to develop. If either of the poles becomes predominant in our life for too long, we will then experience the other afterwards all the more intensely. However, as a result of experiencing the second pole more vividly, our movement back into life will become more profound.

In spite of all this, we're all afraid of pain. Perhaps this is because it reminds us of the first farewell we experienced in life—the departure from the womb. Perhaps it's because pain is intrinsically bound up with our fear of losing ourselves and having to be separated... or maybe it's because it reminds us of the difficulty of growth and further development.

I would suggest the pain of labour and birth takes us back to our original experience of pain, to our deep-seated (developmentally linked) fears, to those forgotten 'existential questions' (Who am I? Why am I here?), to *fundamental* questions, all of which we try to forget about in our everyday lives.

Labour pain also reactivates the pain we ourselves experienced during our own birth.

Fear plays an important role in the experience of pain. It is a form of extreme emotional and physical tension and triggers in us the instinct to run away because it is related to the fight-flight system.

THE NATURE OF THE FEAR OF CHILDBIRTH

Fear is an important mechanism in evolutionary terms because it allows us to defend ourselves and protect ourselves from injury. It is basically an instinctive feeling, the perception of a direct and immediate threat, which sends our whole organism into a state of readiness and tension, so that we can deal with the threat. Fear constricts your mind and perception and its goal is self-preservation. All your body's sphincters become tense, so as to ward off the attack, and—for the same reason—your skeletal musculature tenses up so that it is ready for either 'fight' or 'flight'. In other words, your sympathetic nervous system becomes overstimulated.

Because of your natural human drive for self-protection, you are likely to become fearful during labour. You will sense that your body is under attack and this will put you into a state of alarm. The physiological answer to pain is movement. As birth is a paradoxical process, biological fear speeds up labour and will help you to open up, while social fears can inhibit and stop your labour. Fear will also trigger the fight-flight system and your reactions may include:

- fighting, which in terms of female biology, especially during childbirth, means confronting 'danger' or the problem you are facing, opening up to the child and releasing it. In fact, when faced with stress (which produces a peak of adrenaline at other times), women often produce oxytocin and prolactin instead of adrenaline (Taylor, 2002).
- running away, which in terms of birth means contraction and closure
- becoming unable to do anything, or being paralysed.

Only a being who has no possible means of defending itself, will become totally passive. It is, in fact, possible for a labouring woman who is crippled by fear (throughout the parasympathetic nervous system), to 'abandon' her baby suddenly in a precipitous birth. Normally, though, social fear slows labour down or stops it from progressing at all during the first stage, but it accelerates progress in the second stage by triggering a reflex, which has been called a 'fetus ejection reflex' (Odent, 1987). The reason for this differing function is evolutionary because in both cases the effect is to protect you from danger. When you are in the first stage of labour if a threat presents itself, you and your child are safer if your labour stops and you run away. When you reach the second stage, though, in the face of danger it would actually be safer for you to quickly get your baby born, stick it under your arm and *then* run away!

If you react by 'fighting' (opening up), you would need to know exactly what the 'danger' or problem was, and you would need to feel that you had the 'weapons' or 'tools' you needed in order to cope. If it were not possible for you to find out why you were afraid, and therefore if it were impossible for you to confront your fear, a feeling of diffused, all-encompassing threat would remain. In this case would not be easy for you to know how to focus your energy. Fear without any focused action would cause agitation, i.e. anxiety and fearfulness. Deep-seated fear which cannot be expressed, which is not visible to other people, has a strong influence on labour and birth and can make both of them difficult and risky for your baby. This situation contrasts with a labour which is progressing within known boundaries, with clear reference points. In this case, fears are not so distinct and are more phylogenetic in nature. However, the more alienating the birthing environment is and the less you know about the processes of childbirth, the more you are likely to be afraid.

You need to differentiate between ontogenetic fears resulting from external conditions (your previous experiences, losses suffered and negative stories heard), i.e. social fears, and phylogenetic fears, which are inborn and intrinsically bound up with the process of you becoming a human being and giving birth, i.e. these are your biological fears, which are common to all women.

Phylogenetic fears are fears of the unknown, of the unconscious. They include fear of death (which constitutes a profound form of change), 'losing yourself', fear of abandonment, fear of annihilation, fear of life and of its polar dynamics (which include suffering), fear of separation and fear of loss of personal integrity. These fears are felt by all women in all cultures. Only the way in which women deal with their fears differs.

Behind the common ontogenetic fears you experience when you are pregnant, you may often have a hidden deep-lying question and/or an unexpressed need. You may experience many of these fears and they may conceal different things:

- Fear of loss of your personal and physical integrity may conceal your fear of injury (episiotomy, tearing, having stitches), fear of new physical and emotional experiences, fear of 'otherness', fear of your own body changing, or even fear of not being accepted by your partner (i.e. fear of the person you love).
- Fears that your baby may be ill or deformed may conceal fear of the real baby which exists, fear of your own life changing (its rhythm, your interests and your social role). It may conceal a fear of dependency and connection, or a fear of being punished for your own negativity.

- Fear of 'not being perfect', of being inadequate, may conceal fear of becoming a mother, fear of your sexuality, fear of your body itself or your own feelings. It may conceal a lack of faith in your own intuition, a weakness in your social network and a weakness in your relationship with your mother—and of motherhood itself, which is full of conflicting fears.
- Fear of 'what is going to happen' and of pain may conceal your need for respect, your need to know what hospital procedures are and to get to know the staff there... It may conceal your need for intimacy and continuous care from a trusted person, or it may conceal your need for support and encouragement.

When you face the 'battle' of birth in full awareness of its dangers and can boldly take up your 'weapons', you will focus on strategies for coping, not fear

Looking at fears and giving them a name is the first step towards overcoming them. I would like to mention the image of a female warrior, which I use again later, when referring to exercises... When you face the 'battle' of birth in full awareness of its dangers and can boldly take up your 'weapons', you will focus on your strategies for coping and not on your fear.

The physiological link between fear, tension and pain was described very well by Grantly Dick-Read. He said that the more fear is reduced, the more muscular tension and the perception of pain will also be lowered.

The main proponents of the most important historical schools of psycho-prophylaxis say the following about fear...

- **Grantly Dick-Read (1890-1959)**—an obstetrician who promoted an experimental approach, with you in an active role—said that shutting out fear would have the effect of inhibiting your pain. In his opinion, the way to do this was to provide you with information, exercises (body work) and suggestion, as well as loving support during your labour and birth.
- **Leon Chertok (1911-1991)**—a psychiatrist and psychoanalyst who promoted control of pain, with you in a passive role—said that your labour pain cannot really be reduced. However, he said that reducing your fear would help to put you in a position where you would be able to cope with sensations better during contractions. He recommended you use distracting breathing techniques, awareness, therapeutic suggestion, as well as control through hypnosis.
- **Sheila Kitzinger (born 1929)**—a social anthropologist who specialises in pregnancy, childbirth and parenting—promotes the idea that you should transcend any pain you experience by means of your sexuality. She says that you, as a typical woman, no longer want to control yourself or prove to the world that you have learnt specific exercises. She therefore recommends that you take a psychosexual approach to your labour and birth. In order for this to be possible both intimacy and freedom will be important.

- **Michel Odent (born in 1930)**— (a surgeon, hospital manager, researcher and midwife)—emphasises the role of your immediate environment and sees you actively interacting with your environment. He says the external environment will constantly affect the level of stress (fear) you experience. An environment which is full of stimuli will increase your stress and pain, while an intimate environment will reduce your stress, fear and also pain. He recommends that you sing during your pregnancy and that you help yourself to behave instinctually by labouring and birthing in an intimate, protected (i.e. private) environment and by using water.

THE ROLE OF STRESS

The effects of chronic stress on your **pregnancy** The stress hormone cortisol crosses over the placenta but is rendered useless by placental enzymes. However, in the case of chronic stress this protective mechanism no longer works effectively.

The effects of stress on the mother and placenta Constriction of your blood vessels results in decreased blood flow to the placenta. The synthesis of placental hormones is inhibited, particularly in the case of oestrogen (which is responsible for enabling up to 50 times more blood to flow into the placenta), progesterone (which means that uterine contractions are weaker) and prostaglandins (which play an important role in maintaining the tone of placental blood vessels). Specific effects are as follows:

- At the beginning of your pregnancy the effect of stress is different from the effect at the end of your pregnancy. In the first two trimesters the placenta is growing faster than your baby and it creates the conditions for your unborn baby's further development.
- In the first two trimesters since stress results in inhibited placental growth, it causes reduced symmetry and general restricted growth for your baby.
- In the third trimester stress leads to a deficiency in blood flow into the placenta and this causes asymmetrical growth restriction of some of your baby's bodily parts. This kind of growth restriction may affect later generations.
- Your own stress can cause general symptoms in your sympathetic nervous system (agitation, anxious feelings of unrest, superficiality, wakefulness, hyperactivity, dryness in your mucous membranes, stronger contractions of your uterus, etc.).
- Your immune system is weakened as a result of a reduction in T-lymphocytes and protein synthesis, and also a reduction in antibodies and reduced functioning of the lymphocytes and white blood corpuscles. Lymphocytes themselves might produce adrenocorticotropic hormone (ACTH), which increases catecholamines. The production of endorphins and somatotropins is also inhibited.

The baby is not protected from the effect of chronic stress

Effects of emotional stress in your pregnancy

	Low stress	Medium stress	High stress
Prematurity	4%	17%	16.5%
Difficult labour	12.7%	17%	25%
Health problems in the newborn	4.2%	12.5%	13.8%
Newborn difficulties (reflux, colic, vomiting)	9.4%	13.8%	37.5%
Very demanding children (with sleep disturbances, feeding problems, painful hiccups)	31.6%	50%	76%

(Adapted from Relier, 1994)

The effects of stress on your child Stress causes neuro-immune modulation. In other words, chronic stress influences the primary adaptation system (and therefore damages the thymus gland) (Bottaccioli, 1997). During pregnancy there is symmetrical or asymmetrical growth restriction. After the birth, there is likely to be overactivity, frequent reflux, behavioural abnormalities, illness, etc (Relier, 2001). During pregnancy your growing baby's compensatory mechanisms in distress situations work in the following ways:

- Your baby's haemoglobin levels increase
- There is reduced blood flow on the periphery of your baby's body, in its digestive system, in its liver and in its kidneys.
- There are fewer fetal movements and breathing movements
- Your growing baby's heart rate is reduced and there is an increase in blood flow from its heart.
- Your growing baby experiences fewer REM-phases of sleep; this is problematic because REM sleep is important for the development of its brain.
- In extreme cases, your growing baby's large liver releases blood which is rich in oxygen into the blood circulation

The effects of chronic stress on your experience of the birth itself It is important to differentiate between chronic and acute stress. While acute stress has a stimulating, activating and vitalising effect, and is necessary for your progress in the second stage, chronic stress would be inhibiting and dangerous for both your own and your baby's health.

Photo © Sandro Pintus

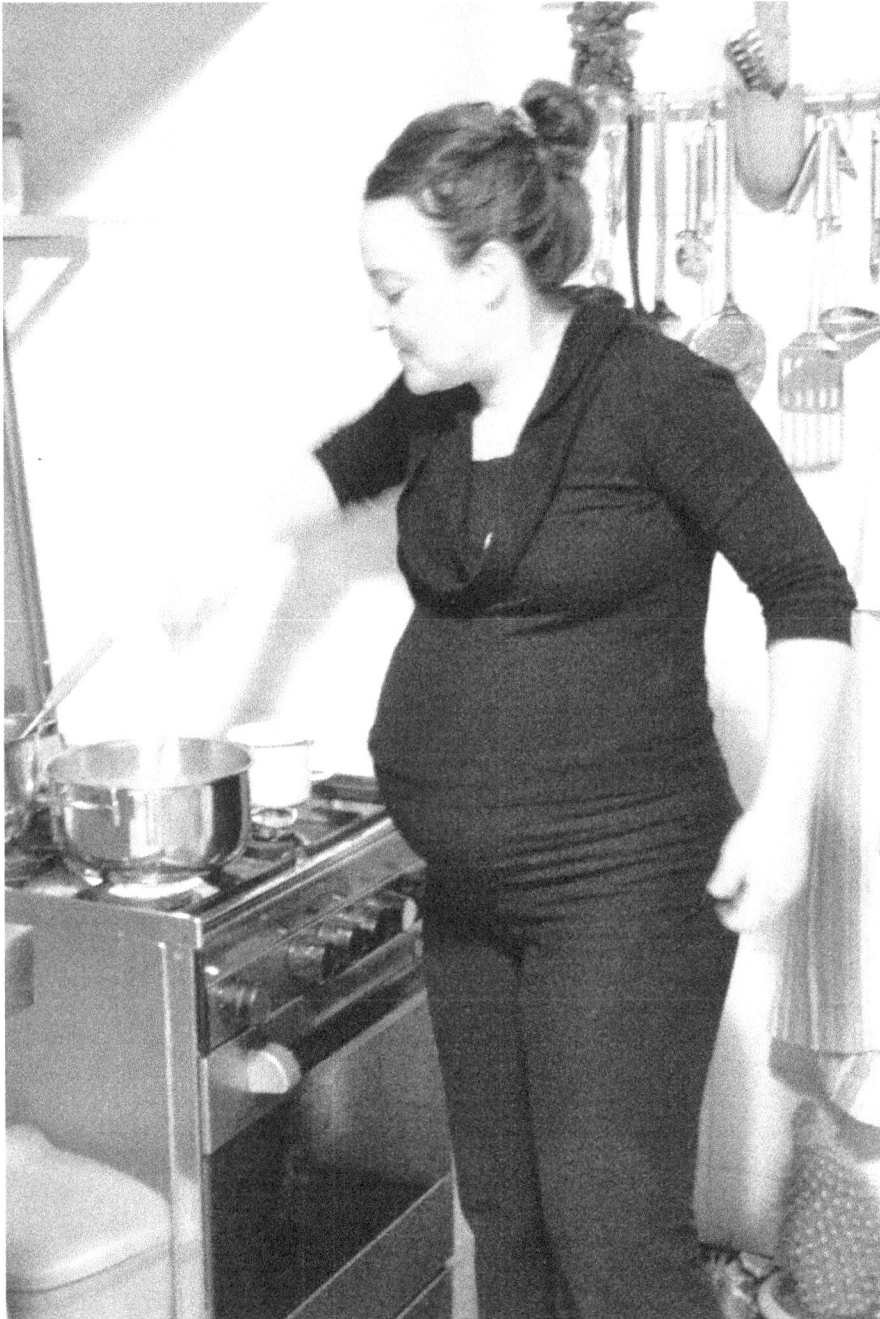

Of course, there can be many causes of stress during pregnancy

If you continuously produce catecholamines, they will stimulate beta-receptors in your flat musculature and they will inhibit its ability to become activated. If you produce catecholamines in a pulsatile way (as in the case of acute stress), they will stimulate your alpha-receptors and thereby increase the responsiveness of your mymetrium. Therefore, what is critical, in terms of the two types of stress, is its rhythm. Acute stress is polar and rhythmical, with high peaks alternating with deep phases of relaxation and feelings of well-being. Chronic stress, by contrast, displays a constant, linear pattern, with hardly any discernible change between tension and relaxation.

The effects on the nature of pain Acute stress will create spasm-like pain which will tend to make you react against the pain—you will feel you can't tolerate it, you are likely to withdraw and close yourself off (and also hold your baby back). The pain itself will tend to become severe, without breaks.

The hormonal and neurophysiological effects of stress This stimulates the continuous production of ACTH, which means you would produce less oxytocin, endorphins and prolactin, and you immune system would be less able to react. The increased tension in your pelvis would have a negative effect on the flow of blood to your uterus. The consequence of this would be that information transmission by hormones and neurotransmitters would also be inhibited.

The different effects on uterine activity Stress causes primary hyperactivity in your uterus. This would make your contractions stronger and the pain worse, and it would cause secondary hypoactivity. Because you would produce less oxytocin, your uterine contractions would become weaker. Alternatively, the effect might be uterine hypertonia, meaning that you would experience strong contractions and be unable to relax in the breaks between contractions, and this would result in persistent pain. The uterus and cervix would stop working together harmoniously, so you would experience failure to progress during the second stage.

The effects on the cervix Your cervix would constrict in a painful, cramp-like way. The lower segment of your uterus would tense up.

The effects on your baby's engagement and the mechanical aspects of birth Increased tension in your pelvis during labour would lead to tension and cramping in your pelvic muscles, which would cause a reduction in the size of your pelvic area. This would make it difficult for your unborn baby's head to engage in your pelvis properly. As a result there would be no significant progress during your labour.

Increased tension in your body would cause a reduction in the size of your pelvic area. This would make it hard for your unborn baby's head to engage in your pelvis.

Tension and the cramping of your uterine muscles would result in distortion of your child's axis with the birth canal. This would lead to asynclitism (i.e. your baby would not get properly positioned in the birth canal) and to a lack of flexion of your baby's head. Tension and cramping of the muscles of your pelvic floor would also result in a reduction in the size of your pelvic area and your pelvic outlet. This would cause back pain, it would prevent rotation of your baby's head, and would lead to various types of malpresentation and deep transverse arrest (when your baby would get stuck in your pelvis). Your pelvic floor would become tense and hard, so the second stage of your labour would be prolonged, it would become more painful (even for your baby) and the fetus ejection reflex would be impossible. Tearing and episiotomy would be likely.

The effects on your internal organs You would retain urine and would probably be unable to pass stools (i.e. you would probably be constipated), and it's likely you would vomit often and for a long time on each bout.

The effects on your placenta See the effects of chronic stress on pregnancy.

The effects on your baby Fetal movements may become first restless, then they would slow down or even stop. Your unborn baby or newborn might experience tachycardia, variable decelerations, inhibited breathing movements and acidosis. At the time of your baby's birth, he or she would probably have breathing problems, as well as difficulty adapting to life outside your womb.

Stress may also result in restless fetal movements, slower movements or none at all. Your baby's vital functions may also be affected in significant ways.

The effects on your own behaviour All kinds of reactions are possible, including wakefulness and over-alertness, restlessness, excitement, resignation or passivity. You may experience anxiety, fear, you may show a tendency to run away or withdraw, or you may constantly ask for help. You may become overly dependent, and may seem to be physically rigid and/or immobile. It's possible you might insist on lying in bed and sleeping (i.e. you might withdraw) or you might claim you were in extreme pain—saying you are experiencing horrific fear.

The clinical signs of chronic stress You may either have a higher basal temperature or you might start shivering. You might look very pale, have dry mucous membranes, and have acidic, strong-smelling sweat. Your eyes might be wide open and look fearful. Your vagina might be constricted, your cervix rigid and you have problems passing urine. You might experience painful fetal movements.

Stress may even cause painful fetal movements

Tools for reducing psychological pain

Writing in 1953, the English obstetrician and author, Grantley Dick-Read spoke about three different ways of exerting an influence, which—in my opinion—are still of relevance today, even if we need to change the content of the teaching. Firstly, there is teaching (and learning), secondly exercises (body work), and thirdly suggestion. Chertok called these same factors education, physiotherapy and psychotherapy (Chertok and Langen, 1962). He felt that it is important for you have a private, intimate environment to labour in, he thought you should know about birth processes and also that you should be able to move around freely during your labour, abandoning your cultural conditioning—if you are to deal with your fear of giving birth.

The view that labour pain needs to be controlled started when men came into the birthing room

From a historical point of view, the idea that labour pain needs to be controlled originated from the time when men started to attend births. On the one hand, male birth attendants had difficulty understanding and accepting the phenomenon of labour pain, and on the other, since labouring women had been brought together in hospitals, it was intolerable having many women in one place, simultaneously experiencing and expressing pain. All experimentation was focused on either eliminating or controlling labour pain. Dick-Read, who spent many hours keeping labouring women company, was the only exception to this trend.

Numerous research studies produced theoretical physiological models of labour pain and the various methods worked with one or other dimension of pain. However, not one method embraced all dimensions. For this reason the application of these methods was only ever partially successful. Nevertheless, you should be optimistic about achieving some positive effects because, as the technique of biofeedback has shown, significant physical changes occur during certain processes—which used to be considered impossible to influence, such as the heart rate, blood pressure and brain waves—so these have now, in fact, been shown to be susceptible to change.

WORKING WITH YOUR FEAR AND TENSION

Dick-Read talked about a fear-tension-pain syndrome. Even he started out with the same preconceptions about birth as was usual at that time, i.e. that labour pain was pathological. He felt that since birth was a natural process it should also be painfree. Dick-Read observed that fear caused tension in the muscles, especially in muscles which 'closed the body off' so as to protect it. He reasoned that the birth canal became constricted in response to fear, and that pain and resistance were the result. He recognised, though, that labouring women were very susceptible to suggestion, which could lead to a state of mind which would involve a loss of memory and a reduction in the amount of pain experienced. Nevertheless, he didn't want to bring women into this state of mind using hypnosis.

He felt that the process of a physiological labour and birth inhibited any kind of rational activity and caused profound psychic and spiritual relaxation. He also thought that women always slipped into a sleepy, dazed state of mind in later stages of labour, when they were not disturbed by fear or anxiety.

Incidentally, it is worth mentioning here that Dick-Read was the first author to outline the importance of the first mother-baby contact. In *Childbirth Without Fear* (Pinter & Martin 2007, originally published in 1959) he explained that even before the baby became separated from the umbilical cord, he would hold the newborn up high so that the mother could see and understand how her dreams had come true. He said his 'patients' were always the first people to hold the newborn baby's little finger and the first to stroke their soft skin and cheeks. As a result, he said that the baby's first cry would be deeply impressed on the new mother's mind as an indelible memory. He felt that there was a profound reason and purpose behind the mother's ecstasy, just as with any of life's other 'grand' feelings, and he felt that the environment was critical at this point in the process. He said that no mother and no newborn baby should be robbed of this mystical relationship.

With reference to muscular relaxation he made another interesting observation. He said that relaxing the whole face is extremely important... Furrowed brows should be avoided! He was convinced that a woman who could relax her face would easily be able to cope with the second stage of labour. In his experience of working with women, though, relaxing the facial muscles was the hardest set of muscles to relax in the whole body. The following points summarise Dick-Read's approach:

- It is essential to eliminate your fear by properly preparing yourself for childbirth. He felt you could achieve this preparation by obtaining information (through teaching/learning), by doing exercises to relax your muscles and by deconditioning your negative thoughts about pain (through the use of suggestion).
- It is necessary for there to be empathy between you and your birth attendant. It is also vital for a midwife to be present all through your labour and birth, so that you have a familiar point of reference, which you feel you trust.

International experiences of Dick-Read's method were very positive. During labour and birth, there were fewer medical problems, a reduced use of drugs, higher tolerance of pain and fewer births ending in a forceps, vacuum or caesarean delivery. After the birth, fewer newborn babies needed rescuscitation, there were fewer cases of postpartum haemorrhage, women seemed happier, their milk production was better and new parents felt more comfortable in their role, and better prepared for the tasks which awaited them. In addition, these experiences showed that although labour pain was not completely eliminated, it was better tolerated and it was possible to reduce it to its physiological minimum. Dick-Read recognised the relationship between pain, emotional experience and strength during childbirth.

PSYCHOPROPHYLAXIS FOR A PAINFREE BIRTH

Psychoprophylaxis (proposed by Nicolaiev in 1949) was a further development and represented a synthesis of various methods which existed around the year 1950. It was based on the assumption that it is possible to eliminate or even prevent labour pain.

METHODS FOR CONDITIONING REFLEXES

These methods also originated in the Russian school of hypnosis. They were based on Pavlov's famous behavioural experiment. He was the person who researched the mechanism of conditioned reflexes using dogs and he later also transferred the same methodology to women preparing for childbirth. The idea was to condition a physiological reaction by training people with a reward.

Velvosky, Vellay and Chertok were the most important proponents of this work. The model of birth which underpinned their method was mechanistic, since it assumed that bodily processes could function in the same way as machines—i.e. that they could be logical and linear.

CONDITIONING METHODS USING SUGGESTION

In 1968 Chertok asserted that 83% of women were so afraid of giving birth that they should have psychotherapy. He believed that labour pain only existed because of negative influences and he denied that physiology could be the cause.

Methods which use suggestion are based on different schools of hypnosis and psychotherapy (e.g. those of Chertok and Lukas). They are also based on the conviction that words can be used to distract women (as Lamaze believed) by activating the neocortex, or that verbal suggestions can be given by a trusted person with whom the labouring woman has a good relationship (as Dick-Read believed). All methods reflect the belief that women were 'deficient' and that correction of this 'deficiency' is necessary, or that the environment is responsible (as Dick-Read proposed).

By 'hypnosis' is meant an altered state of consciousness, which is achieved by numbing the rational mind. This state is achieved using verbal instructions, breathing, distraction or sensory stimulation. Hypnosis was the first scientifically recognised method of natural pain relief.

Trials began in the 19th century in France. In 1819 the Abbé Farria used the words 'lucid sleep' to describe the hypnotic state and hypnosis was used for the first time for a birth in 1833 by Pierre Foissac. He called it 'animal magnetism' since it appeared to put the woman into an 'electromagnetic' sleep. Between 1920-1935 a well-known school of hypnosis operated in Russia, with important researchers such as Platonov, Nicolaiev, Velvosky and many others and this resulted in hypnosis being officially recognised and judged as effective. Taking hypnosis as a starting point, many other methods of *post-hypnotic suggestion* developed. These involved teaching women before they went into labour and offered them an 'anchor', which they could use during labour to put themselves back into a state of hypnosis. Cassette tapes were used which included hypnotists' suggestions, music, instructions for staring at a specific point and, later on, also methods for conditioning reflexes. The woman's state of consciousness was akin to sleep or a half-sleeping state. The modern American school (which started with the work of Peter Blythe, in the 1960s) defines hypnosis as an altered state of consciousness, which makes a person receptive to influence through suggestion and which causes involuntary reactions. Hypnosis is a mental condition in which suggestion can not only easily be made, but in which suggestion becomes much stronger, than it might be in a normal state of mind (Agnetti, 1992). Chertok and Langen define hypnosis as voluntary susceptibility to influence, i.e. emotional influence on the psychic and physical woman through interpersonal contact (Chertok and Langen, 1968).

Practitioners of hypnosis have reported various occurrences, ranging from the complete disappearance of pain to the vague perception of contractions, which weren't painful—and even to women only being able to remember the very last contractions of the second stage of labour. (However, we need to take into account the fact that the hospital births that were described were almost exclusively difficult, pathological births which had many complications.) Hypnosis always seems to have minimised pathology and facilitated a natural outcome for birth. However, at first no expression of pain or emotions from the labouring women themselves was considered. Later studies on hypnosis revealed that vocalisations and spoken words could influence the dynamics in the body and change the physiological processes.

Earlier methods were based on influencing people by distracting them and using suggestion, working with the client's faith in and dependency on the hypnotist. These methods were also based on post-hypnotic suggestion, which made people lose any memory of painful experiences. This worked by disassociating the physiological mechanism of pain on various levels and largely blocking any behavioural expression of pain. This method makes the woman passive and she goes into a sleepy state of mind. However, blocking an experience which is as highly charged as childbirth may well cause depression and inhibit other physiological processes, such as breastfeeding.

Nevertheless, experiments with hypnosis helped people recognise certain important aspects of labour pain. They revealed the psychic components of labour pain and the enormous importance of attitude towards pain, as well as the role of empathetic behaviour of birth attendants towards the woman in labour and giving birth (which relates to the affective–motivational dimension). Further developments in hypnotic methods focused on one or other of these technical aspects. It was only later that people proposed that the labouring woman use active self-hypnosis in an awake state of mind.

Experiments with hypnosis helped people recognise certain important aspects of labour pain

Classical hypnosis works on the sensory-perceptive dimension of pain, which is separate from the affective-motivational dimension. Hypnosis involves suggestion, which prevents the perception and evaluation of pain stimuli and it is supposed to also dissolve conscious memory. While it is taking place, the labouring woman remains passive. With this kind of hypnosis, the intensive stimulation of pain stimuli is stopped, but no opportunity is provided to remove the stimuli. They are therefore likely to remain a subconscious burden in the physiological system.

A subconscious burden may be left in the system

In my own clinical practice I have seen cases of postnatal depression and breastfeeding problems after women have used hypnosis for labour. Another disadvantage of hypnosis is that it needs to be practised regularly and often demands the presence of a hypnotist during labour and birth. After all, hypnosis is essentially a form a psychotherapy so it should only be used by specialists who are trained in its use.

On the positive side, according to Milton Erikson, modern hypnosis constitutes a natural mental process, which facilitates natural mental mechanisms (Erickson, 1967). This may well be the case but birth hormones bring the woman into a state of hypnosis in a spontaneous way. A hypnotic state induced by a hypnotist, on the other hand, always involves an increased susceptibility to suggested behavioural changes and the changed behaviour may not always be helpful in terms of facilitating labour and birth.

In fact, naturally induced hypnotic states are very likely to occur in labour, thanks to the extremely strong influence of the parasympathetic nervous system during pregnancy and labour. In physiological terms women are particularly receptive to speech involving imagery, to trances and spontaneous states of hypnosis. As a result, every midwife should understand how to communicate at this level. By using appropriate choices of words and gentle suggestion, your midwife can help you improve your health during pregnancy and help you to either reduce your pain, or accept it. Suggestions from your midwife can also free you from your negative conditioning and help you to see the positive aspects of what you experience. (This relates to the cognitive–evaluating dimension.) Active self-hypnosis is one method (among others) which your midwife can use to decondition your cultural and personal negative imprinting. It will leave intact your channels for expressing and unloading pain. In this case, suggestion works primarily by helping you to tolerate pain, i.e. it works on the affective-motivational dimension.

But how does it work in practice? During labour a natural change in consciousness seems to take place when the physiological processes are proceeding undisturbed and your perception will change. This seems to be an indispensible physiological process which allows your cervix to fully dilate, your pain to be reduced and spontaneous birth to occur.

Hormones, especially endorphins, and the powerful collective stimulation and dominance of your archaic brain cause beta brain waves to slow down to become alpha waves, and then, when you are in active labour, these will even transmute into theta waves. This slowing down of your brain waves will increase your ability to synchronise processes, they will sharpen your sensory perceptions, and also your perception of emotions. As a result, you will become very sensitive and receptive to suggestion and to outside influences. According to Melzak, deep meditation, intensive concentration and observation of feelings, sensations or inner images can bring you to a state of mind which is very similar to the hypnotic state used for pain relief (Melzak, 1973). Every word and every gesture seems particularly significant at this time and is likely to indelibly influence your perception of things while you are in labour .

This hypnotic state will reach its highest point when you are in transition—i.e. between the first and second stages of your labour. You will lose all your inhibitions and behave very instinctively—some would say like an *animal*. Your ways of expressing yourself verbally and physically will become very assertive and you may experience (and later describe) the pain of labour more as power and intense feeling... while the suffering aspect of the pain will fade into the background.

The degree of exhaustion and the feeling of having no more energy left, which you may experience at this time, will prepare you for complete surrender, or it would be a sign that this had already occurred. You are very likely to give up and say something like, "I can't do it any more!" and demand some kind of pain relief, a caesarean or something else, so that you can escape from this situation. You might even say: "Let's just go home and come back again tomorrow!" If, at this point, your midwife or your partner share this feeling of capitulation and helplessness, you will tend not to react appropriately in terms of your real needs (so as to give birth successfully). In other words, this is the only moment during a labour and birth when your midwife or partner shouldn't respond to your requests because this behaviour would represent a turning point.

During labour by speaking in a way which is rich in imagery, symbols and archetypes, or even better through silence and positive gestures and other body language your midwife can directly communicate with you and positively influence you. Using symbolic, colourful and positive words she may be able to advise you. If she were to ask you to listen to reason or if she were to disturb your environment, your labour would slow down or stop any you wouldn't make any further progress. If she just waits, in a very short time you will find new resources and strength within yourself and unexpectedly discover new capabilities. You will get a second wind which will prepare you for a feeling of joy at the time of the birth. My view, based on my own experience of attending women in labour for over 30 years, is that if your midwife were to interrupt you or try and change this phase of the birthing process then she would be robbing you of this powerful experience.

PHYSIOLOGICAL METHODS

These methods were developed between 1930-1954 by Jacobsen and were based on progressive relaxation of the muscles. The idea was to send inhibiting information to the intrathalamic vegetative and extrapyramidal nuclei in the brain. This concept was entirely mechanical and rational, since Jacobsen dismissed the role of hypnotic suggestion, as well as the role of a personal relationship for achieving a relaxed state. For him, relaxation was a passive process involving doing nothing. In other words, it was a technique, which—through practice—could be learnt.

Relaxation was seen as a passive technique to be learnt

To Jacobsen it was meaningless for there to be a personal relationship between the woman and her attendant(s). He believed that it was not a good idea to encourage pregnant women to be enthusiastic about the mechanisms of birth, or to help them to understand them. He felt that in doing so there was the risk of strengthening pregnant women's emotional reactions.

His methods were not widely used, but the physiological rule on which they were based became part of psychoprophylaxis.

AUTOGENIC TRAINING AND CLASSICAL PSYCHOPROPHYLAXIS

In the case of autogenic training, breathing techniques are linked to relaxation. The long out-breath is considered an important tool for releasing tension, inhibiting the neocortex and increasing sensitivity to suggestion.

Psychoprophylaxis was a combination between autogenic training and the methods of suggestion. Its various proponents used slightly different methods, but followed similar principles. Velvosky (a Soviet psychologist) prepared women using a purely cognitive approach, then during contractions in labour they were supposed to breathe slowly and deeply, while counting from 1 to 10, in order to distract themselves from the pain. In the breaks between contractions he put no emphasis on relaxation. Lamaze (a French obstetrician, who developed his ideas in the 1940s) preferred deep breathing alternating with fast, light breathing and panting at the crest of each contraction and during transition and second stage. His goal was also to distract women and stimulate the neocortex. Suzanne Arms described this method (in 1975) as being a way of changing birth from being a means of making deep contact with one's own body, to being a means of distracting oneself. Lamaze didn't see any purpose in getting women to relax in the breaks between contractions.

In general, in all these methods relaxation is only seen as being useful during contractions. The gradual build-up of physical exercises which Dick-Read considered important (which some people today would call 'body work') was not a part of psychoprophylactic birth preparation.

Discussions about the effectiveness and limitations of psychoprophylaxis revolve around a physiological contradiction... In order to make the woman receptive to suggestion, it is necessary to reduce the activity of the neocortex. Nevertheless, in psychoprophylaxis in order to achieve pain relief during labour through distraction, the activity of the neocortex was stimulated, through distraction—because proponents of psychoprophylasixis believed this was how the physiological centralised spread of pain could be suppressed. Many authors emphasise the necessity of reducing the activity of the neocortex during pregnancy for relaxation, but they give the contradictory advice that the cerebral neocortex should be stimulated during labour, so as to achieve pain relief through distraction and suggestion.

Psychoprophylaxis involves a contradiction... It's not possible to reduce the activity of your neocortex and stimulate it at the same time so as to distract you.

Given this contradiction, it's easy to understand why psychoprophylaxis can be effective in the early (latent) stages of labour, while the neocortex is still active. However, when a woman is in active labour either distraction simply stops working as a method of pain relief, or it causes labour to slow down.

A big disadvantage of psychoprophylaxis lies in the fact that it presents itself as a method which can stand alone. Its simplification into the method which calls itself the 'The RAT Method' or 'respiratory autogenic training' has even been patented and claims to be useful for all kinds of people. (It is a method which is used on a widespread basis in Italy, with midwives taking a short course to learn it. The British Autogenic Society promotes its use in the UK.) If there is any advantage in this method at all, it is probably that in learning it many women come together and therefore have the opportunity to make contact with each other and learn a bit about themselves. Then again, this linear method creates expectations about birth and women consequently make demands on themselves... but the method has a high failure rate, so women are almost always disappointed afterwards. This is partly because the method does not look at a woman as an individual or as a whole person; it is also because the method is based on the contradictory goals mentioned before, which are in conflict with the nature of childbirth.

In fact, this method has produced the image of the 'perfect birthing woman', who can bring her pain under control. Her reaction to the pain she experiences (not only on a physiological level but also as a result of medical intervention) has to be silent and well-adapted. Clearly, this is not realistic.

The image of the perfect birthing woman is not realistic

PSYCHOSEXUAL METHODS

Sheila Kitzinger considers childbirth to be an important part of female sexuality within the life cycle of every woman. She emphasises the meaningful, sexual and emotional aspects of childbirth and breastfeeding, without denying their painful aspects. She maintains that you must learn to trust your body and your own instincts, so that you can have a deeply moving, holistic experience of birth (Kitzinger, 1985).

Her method of antenatal preparation aims to help you become self-reliant, help you get in touch with yourself, help you exercise freedom of choice, help you develop the ability to assert your wishes to your birth attendants and— above all—help you become aware of your own freedom. She believes that when you have the freedom to decide yourself, where, how and with whom you give birth this is a question of power and lack of oppression, of freedom and sexual autonomy. Finally, like Odent, Kitzinger emphasises the importance of you having an intimate, undisturbed environment for childbirth.

ACTIVE, HOLISTIC METHODS

With these methods we are not talking about one single model of pain management or relief, but about various kinds of preparation for labour and birth. These methods include self-hypnosis, yoga, bioenergy, watzu (i.e. preparing to give birth in water), prenatal singing, and preparation for birth as a life experience, among others. With all these methods there is the idea of making you more active so that you can take control of birth as much as possible. The goal is to help you to accept labour and birth pain as a unique opportunity for personal development, to express this pain and thereby see birth as a value-free experience, however it turns out to be. Each approach has developed in different places, probably over millennia, and none of them can really be said to have originated with any particular proponents, although certain people have certainly encouraged the use of one or another method at different points in time. For example, Michel Odent became well-known in the 1970s as a doctor (who was working as an obstetrician) who advocated the use of these methods. In the early 1980s Janet Balaskas published her thoughts on the importance of making birth *active* in the book *Active Birth* (Unwin, 1983) republished later as *New Active Birth* (Harvard Common Press, 1994). She continued to promote active, holistic methods from that time onwards, by founding the Active Birth Centre in London (find out more at www.activebirthcentre.com).

All active and holistic methods are based on the hypothesis that in order for your labour to progress it is important for your neocortex to be inhibited. The altered state of consciousness which you experience when your neocortex is inhibited is a necessary physiological foundation for everything else. You will seem to become more tolerant of pain if you are motivated, if you remain active (on an instinctual level), and if you use the breaks between contractions to relax. When you move around during contractions your tensions will seem to dissipate.

In these active approaches to birth preparation, the acceptance of pain is a central theme. This is because pain is seen as being an indispensible component of a conscious birthing experience and it is interpreted as being part of your strength while you are in labour. The important physiological function of pain is recognised.

As part of these active approaches you are given all possible information, so that you can fearlessly make decisions, including about the kinds of pain relief you would like to use so as to reduce pain to its physiological minimum (if you opt to have a physiological birth), or about the drug-based pain relief you would like to use—although, of course, you would then become inactive.

In order to inhibit your neocortex and stimulate your primary brain, instead of emphasising the transmission of knowledge, emphasis is placed on intuition. Instead of suggesting ways for you to behave, you are encouraged to follow your instincts, and do what you feel you need to do in order to fulfil your needs.

Despite the development of many active, holistic methods, and even the acceptance that they are a valid approach, in many antenatal courses, you may find you are still being prepared to be obedient and submissive and to follow your 'unchangeable' destiny. The information you receive from midwives and other birth attendants may often be incomplete and filtered. You will be expected to trust your 'care team' (in other words, delegate all responsibility to these people) and rely on them. To undermine your expectations before labour and your efforts when it actually begins, you may well be offered drug-based pain relief and many caregivers will expect you to need it.

In fact, while you are in labour, if you say you want to experience birth fully consciously and deal with pain using your own resources, your caregivers should just encourage you in all good conscience when all important conditions relating to your environment are fully met. This means that you should have intimacy, freedom of movement and the freedom to express yourself as you wish. This is because, in my experience, it is only in these conditions that the physiological reactive mechanisms to pain function properly.

Your midwives should create these conditions, at least if you ask for them. Nowadays no caregiver can justify forcing you to endure excessive pain during labour and birth caused by an unsupportive environment or by medical interventions. After all, this would represent a form of violence towards you, because there certainly are other possibilities.

If we weigh up cost versus effectiveness and quality assurance issues, the question remains as to whether it is a good idea for hospitals to continue investing in drug-based methods of pain relief and the medico-technical model of birth. We should consider whether it would make more sense, instead, to invest in providing an environment which would facilitate the physiology of birth, and invest in midwives who are trained in how to provide personal support for women experiencing the natural, physiological processes. Whatever the answer to this question, all options should be available to you.

If we attempted to get to the heart of the issue of pain during labour and birth by examining all key factors, we would perhaps not conclude that any one particular method is best, but would choose that comprehensive provision be available, which would cater to women's individual needs. Midwives need to use many types of physiological methods, but the most important thing must always be to focus on you while you're in labour and giving birth. You yourself must experiment and discover your own deep needs.

For this to be possible it is important for you to find out about the fears you harbour, based on your experiences in life, or on what you have heard and then deal with your negative imprinting. You need to be motivated to do this and you need to appreciate the existential issues which arise around labour and birth pain. By experiencing the pain of labour and birth you will have a unique opportunity to deepen your experience of life and promote your own further development. Doing this will involve working particularly on the affective-motivational dimension and the cognitive-evaluating dimension of pain.

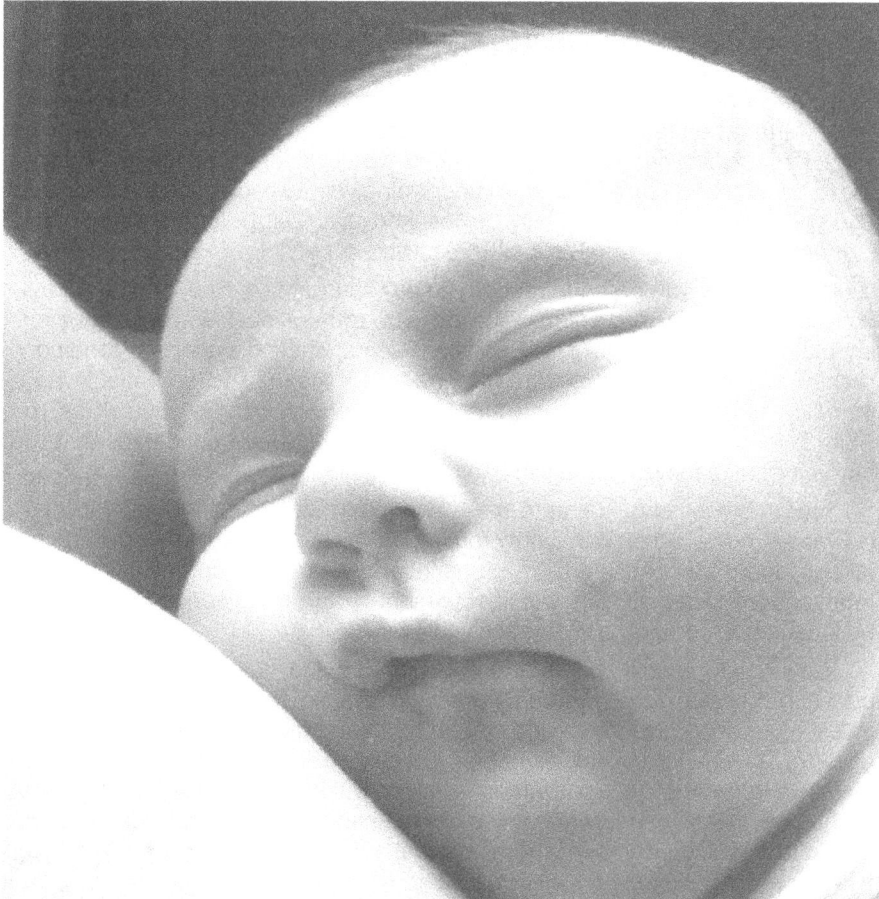

It's interesting to consider what the difference might be for your baby during labour...

A comparison between psychoprophylaxis and active methods

Psychoprophylaxis	Active methods
Labour pain is not natural	Labour pain is natural and to be accepted
Labour must be controlled	You must surrender and let yourself go
You must be rational and have an active neocortex	You need to let yourself open up from within and behave instinctually
Rhythms are linear, flat and static	Rhythms are variable, individual, penetrative
You mustn't express any pain or fear	You must be free to express any pain and fear
You need to inhibit the mechanisms which prompt you to physiologically react to pain	You need to support the mechanisms which prompt you to react physiologically to pain
You need to be passive	You need to be active
You need to be trained in a method	You need to experiment with your own resources and use your own experience
You need to apply a 'technique' when you give birth	You need to behave instinctively and spontaneously
You need to limit your behaviour	You can behave in many different ways
You must be motivated to use the method	You must be motivated to experience childbirth
The baby is not an active part of the birthing process	The baby is seen as an active part of the birthing process
You need to use learnt, rehearsed knowledge while you're in labour	When you are in labour you need to use all levels of dynamic knowledge
You need to relax during contractions	You need to relax during the breaks between contractions
You need to remain still	You can move around freely and be active
You need to achieve muscular relaxation by concentrating on relaxing	You need to achieve muscular relaxation by moving around
You need to try to be a perfect birthing woman	You are the key player in the process and you arrange the birth in your own individual way
You can learn how to give birth and you can succeed or fail at it	Giving birth is an individual and instinctive experience, which will strengthen you, however you experience it
You need to be a perfect, adapted labouring and birthing woman	Your freedom and your individual choice are the most important aspects of labour and birth

RELAXATION EXERCISES

Relaxation exercises can make you feel confident and self-assured and they can help you find your own ways of doing things. They can help you to rediscover your archaic knowledge of how to give birth. These exercises, which you can build into your daily routine, should give you a sense of well-being, they should give you strength and energy and they should help you to develop your own way of communicating. This in turn will allow you to make good contact with your growing baby.

Relaxation exercises draw tension out of your body and open you up so you can improve your state of mind and feel more at peace with yourself. They activate the creative, right side of your brain and inhibit activity in the rational, left side of your brain. In this way an energy flow is achieved from the left side of your brain to the right side, and doing this will restrain any tendency you have to reason and be critical. It is then possible for a midwife or other supportive birth partner to make direct contact with your unconscious and embed positive suggestions into your mind—or you can do this on your own. Your intuition and instincts will be strengthened and your imagination will be stimulated.

Doing these exercises will also allow you to programme yourself positively about childbirth, to a certain extent, and prepare yourself to separate from your baby and face the pain of labour. As a result, during labour, you will be able to behave autonomously. There are many different relaxation techniques, active and passive ones. Trying out various methods is helpful so that you can find the techniques which work best for you.

During labour you will need to quickly relax at the end of every contraction so that the breaks between contractions can be used to restore your strength and so that the production of endorphins can be stimulated. Labour involves constant change between activity (during contractions) and relaxation (during the breaks between contractions). So as to make this fast change easier, you can create a kind of 'anchor' for yourself. This means linking something— an internal image, a sound, calming music, a pleasant aroma or a lovely feeling—with relaxation. With a little practice you will then be able to use this 'anchor' to quickly bring youself back into a state of deep relaxation.

VISUALISATION

This causes the strongest activation of inner resources, including the activation of your archaic knowledge, which all women have, as well as of the parasympathetic nervous system, which has also been called an 'inner wound healer'. Visualisation will free you from your prejudices and negative conditioning. It will allow you to transform your positive thoughts into dynamic mental pictures and these pictures will transform the physiological dynamics of your body. (As I mentioned before, biofeedback has confirmed that this is the case.) In short, visualisation exercises can help you make personal decisions which meet your real, deep needs. They can also help you learn how to speak your feelings directly and have a dialogue with your growing baby.

I refer here to deep visualisations when working in the dimension of the water element, which I explain later, in Chapter 6. As you will see, these are not really guided visualisations, but they can be led with a few archetypal images. These visualisations seem to allow your archaic brain to be stimulated... the place which is your deepest source of energy. By getting in touch with this part of your brain, you can find resources and tools, which will allow you to face the pain of labour.

CULTURAL DECONDITIONING

This is a tool which may be explored during antenatal classes or which you may be able to develop through reading widely about childbirth. It involves working on the cognitive-evaluating dimension. In order to understand your cultural imprinting as it relates to pain, your preconceptions about birth and the type of care you think you need, it is necessary to obtain a historical perspective, and consider the history of childbirth provision and the history of women over the centuries. You need to understand the different values women have put on birth, as well as social and institutional values, and you also need to do some detective work to understand the rituals and protocols which were typical in hospitals at various points in the past. This is how you will gain a better understanding of your 'inner geography', i.e. the nature of the various female images which are embedded inside you. You will then also more clearly understand and acknowledge your own difficulties and ambivalence, as well as your real needs as a woman. It should help you to become aware of your internal and external contradictions and learn about your limitations and potential. It's good if you can freely discuss your numerous imprinted ideas, throw off your emotional baggage and thereby free up your limbic system.

By taking a look at the history of women and the institutions which dealt with birth in the past, you should also understand why institutions object to natural, spontaneous birth and you will be able to choose what seems to be good and useful to you.

It is only when you fully understand your own point of view that you will be able to focus on an objective, which you really want to achieve. Your expectations will then be more realistic and less idealistic.

PERSONAL DECONDITIONING

This is the process by which you analyse and diffuse your own past experiences of pain. You need to talk about your experiences of pain with other women and discuss your fears, which you will become aware of when you tell and listen to stories which were told by mothers, friends and sisters. You can then reflect on what has helped you cope with pain so far and also what *might* have helped you. Even focusing on how you yourself were born can help you better understand your own view of pain, your needs and what resources and types of support are available to you.

You analyse and diffuse your own past experiences

As a woman you will inevitably have a great deal of direct, frequent contact with the subject 'pain'. Whether it's because of your own physiology (menstrual pain, labour pain, pain resulting from loss, for example, from miscarriage, sick children, etc.) or whether it's because you often help out with people who are suffering—or even because of your emotional way of behaving—you probably have a lot more to do with pain than men do. Despite this, you will probably not be keen to discuss this topic and even your birth attendants are likely to shy away from talking about it in depth. Perhaps you are afraid of simply talking about suffering and your birth attendants might be afraid that doing so—getting you to confront your pain and that of others—might push you to a crisis point. Nevertheless, it really is helpful to focus on the physiology of pain and the fear of pain and talk about something that we all face. In doing so, inner tensions are dissolved, instead of being increased. After recognising and defining your fears, you will be able to explore appropriate means of support, in order to overcome them. It is actually *talking about pain* which terrifies many pregnant women and birth attendants the most... Is that true for you too?!

Is it actually talking about pain which terrifies you?!

Many women are afraid they will be 'beside themselves' or that they will no longer know themselves when they express pain. They are afraid of losing control and try to 'master' themselves. Nevertheless, expressing pain and naming fears are both important methods of natural pain relief, because they involve the release of tension in the central brain.

SHARING YOUR EXPERIENCE WITH OTHER WOMEN

Simply getting together with other women—at an antenatal class, for example—has a therapeutic effect and can contribute to the release of tension. Sharing your experiences, you will have many opportunities to free yourself of negative imprinting and conditioning, particularly when you make contact with other women who have already had positive birthing experiences.

BECOMING MOTIVATED AND TAKE AN ACTIVE APPROACH

In every labour it seems that there is some choice, although having only a certain amount of choice is not enough. Even when there is a *little* choice you need to force yourself to make use of your freedom to make choices. You must, at the very least, decide whether you are going to have an active or a passive birth; whether it's going to be a natural or a technological birth; whether it's going to be a birth which uses medical pain relief or none. In our world of 'either-or', in which there are only two possibilities, it is always difficult to make a *real choice.* If women were to follow their real needs, instead of an ideology, much of the time the choice would have to be "I'll have this, as well as that..." The curvaceous number 'three' (3) symbolises this integration of possibilities. Sometimes, in an institutional context, where the offer is 'either... or', you will need to negotiate your needs and ask for more integration.

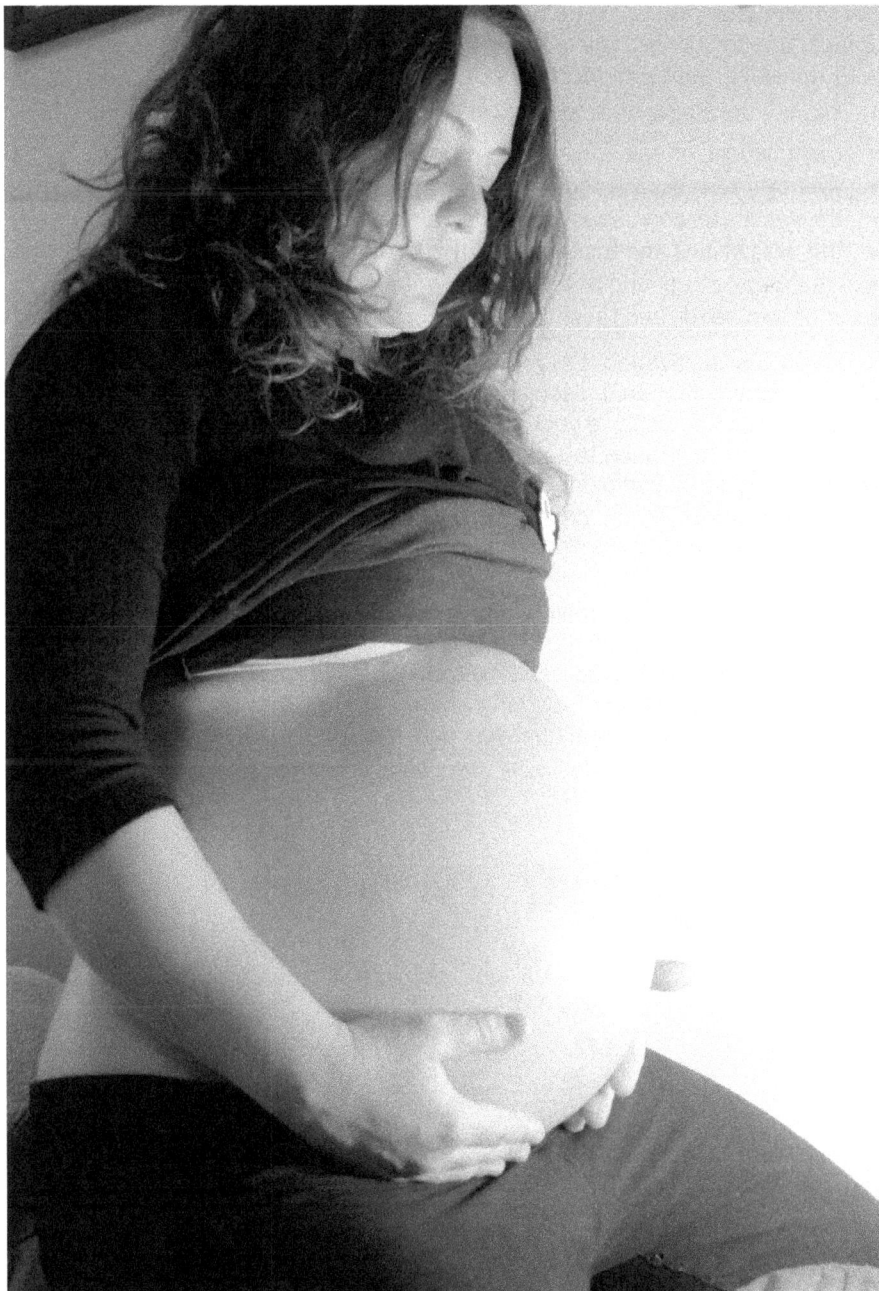

Even when there's only a small element of choice, you need to make the effort to use it

If you want to opt for 'this, as well as that' you will be forced to come to terms with your needs. Only when you have a clear idea of what you want, will you be able to succeed to achieve that, unless you either want to be in conflict with yourself or with your birth attendants.

You will develop a clear idea of what you want when you understand:

- the functions of pain
- your own past experience of pain
- the necessary conditions to reduce pain to its physiological minimum
- the possibilities and tools you can use to deal with pain
- your own cultural and personal conditioning
- your own needs and those of your unborn baby

When your motivation—i.e. your idea of the kind of birth you want—is based on an awareness of your deep-seated, authentic needs, you will actively and effectively work to achieve your goals. This will affect your behaviour, first and foremost. Your tolerance to procedures and interventions will rise even when you don't agree they should be used, as long as your fundamental needs are not compromised. When you really understand your own needs, you will be able to make real choices and accept their positive and negative implications and still hold on to what is important for you.

Establishing what you really want is possible on a rational level (of analysis and knowledge), as well as in the affective-motivational dimension, using physical exercises (as discussed below). When talking about 'learning' it is therefore not a question of learning about anatomy and physiology... Instead, it's to do with working out how you can move into the centre of your own experience so as to discover your own body's knowledge and strengthen its activity.

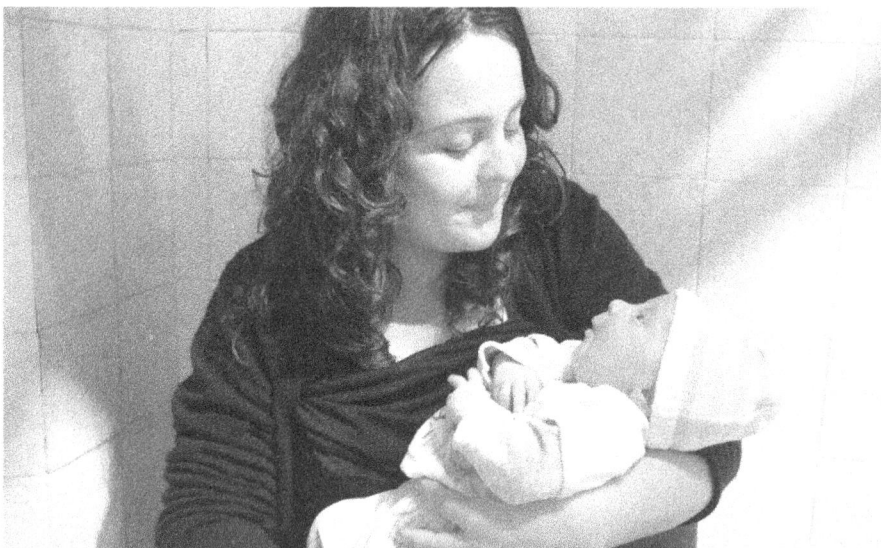

Photo © Sandro Pintus

During labour make sure you're in a totally private environment so you can feel free with your partner

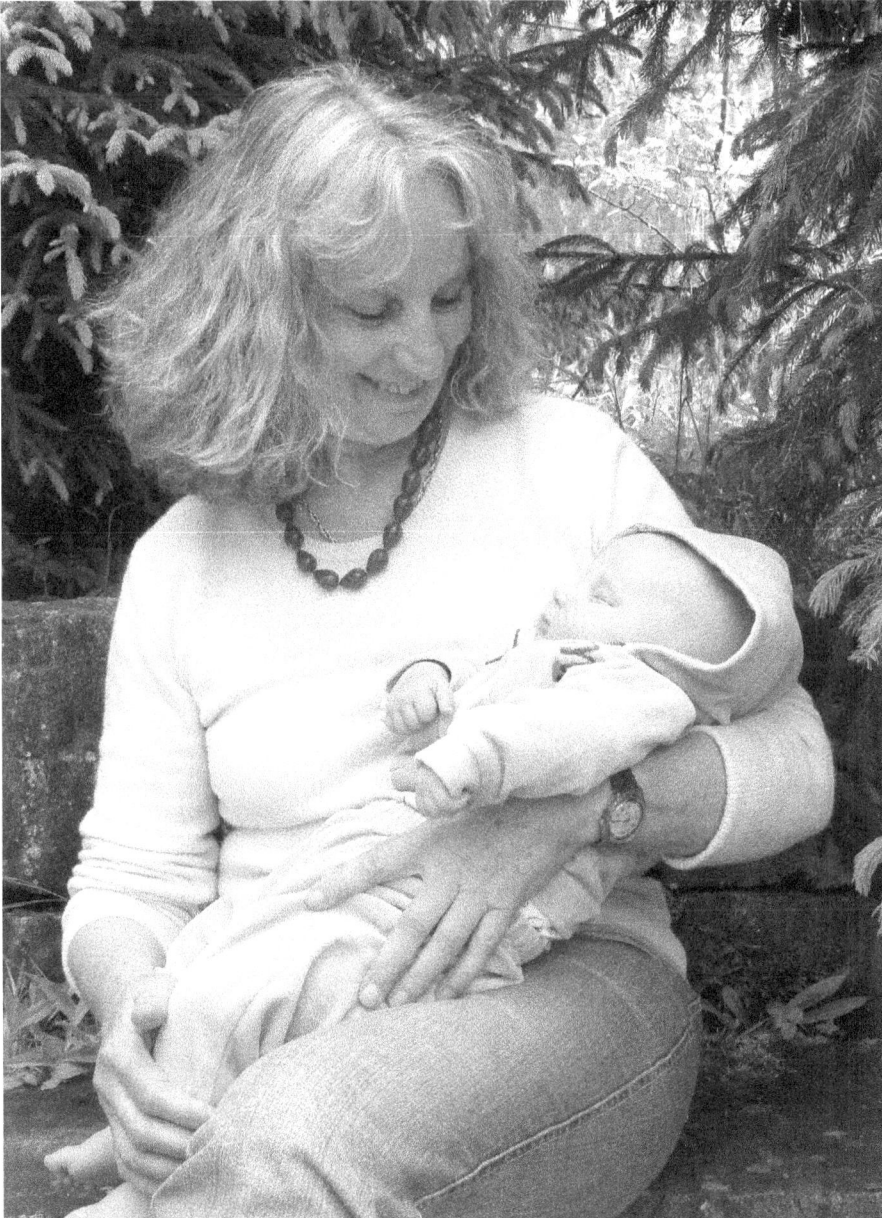

When a baby is conceived of love, it makes sense that its birth should also be characterised by love and tender support. Here Verena cradles her granddaughter. Left: The same baby has a cuddle with his mother.

Exercises (body work)

Physical exercises primarily have two goals:

- **To prepare you for labour and birth in physical terms**
  Tense muscles and lack of flexibility stimulate your reticular system in a negative way. Your neocortex is put into a state of alarm and its sensitivity to the increasing peripheral triggers increases. This means that a much stronger reaction (to pain) follows. By contrast, working the muscles naturally, with relaxed muscle tone, will stimulate your brain structures positively. The inhibiting mechanisms to increasing afferent pain pathways will become activated.

- **To provide you with physical experiences**
  This will allow you to explore your subconscious channels of the birthing process and get to know yourself better. This in turn will mean that you can later activate your own resources. Exercises make experiences concrete and doing them encourages you to experiment, so that you can discover your own best coping strategies. The exercises you do should be very varied and not be limited to just one type of exercise or one technique.

After you do any exercises, it's important to talk about your experiences. Talking about what you've done and the experiences you've had will help you to bring your experimentation and 'practice' into the your *conscious experience*, so that you can use your new skills later.

The importance of continuous emotional support

It's very important to get continuous support during all phases of your pregnancy, labour and birth because it will help to facilitate the physiological processes and effect natural pain relief during your labour. It is now widely accepted that a process of emotional opening up is only possible in a humane and protected environment, because it is only then that you will feel safe and secure. If you have a good, loving relationship with your partner, your most important form of support could be from him because he is emotionally closest to you, he knows you well, he knows from your shared sexual experience how to help you open up and he should be able to keep you grounded in a loving way—so his presence may well constitute the best form of support.

While you're labour you will also need to be aware of how your partner is behaving and will need to consider whether or not he is really fulfilling your needs in the specific situations you find yourself. Sometimes he may not be able to tune into the very female dimension of childbirth, but your midwife may be able to help him do this. In any case you need to make sure you are in a very private environment during your labour because then you will be able to be as intimate and as emotional as you like. In a really private atmosphere, your partner should also start behaving intuitively towards you.

Opening up will only be possible in a humane and protected environment—when you feel safe and secure

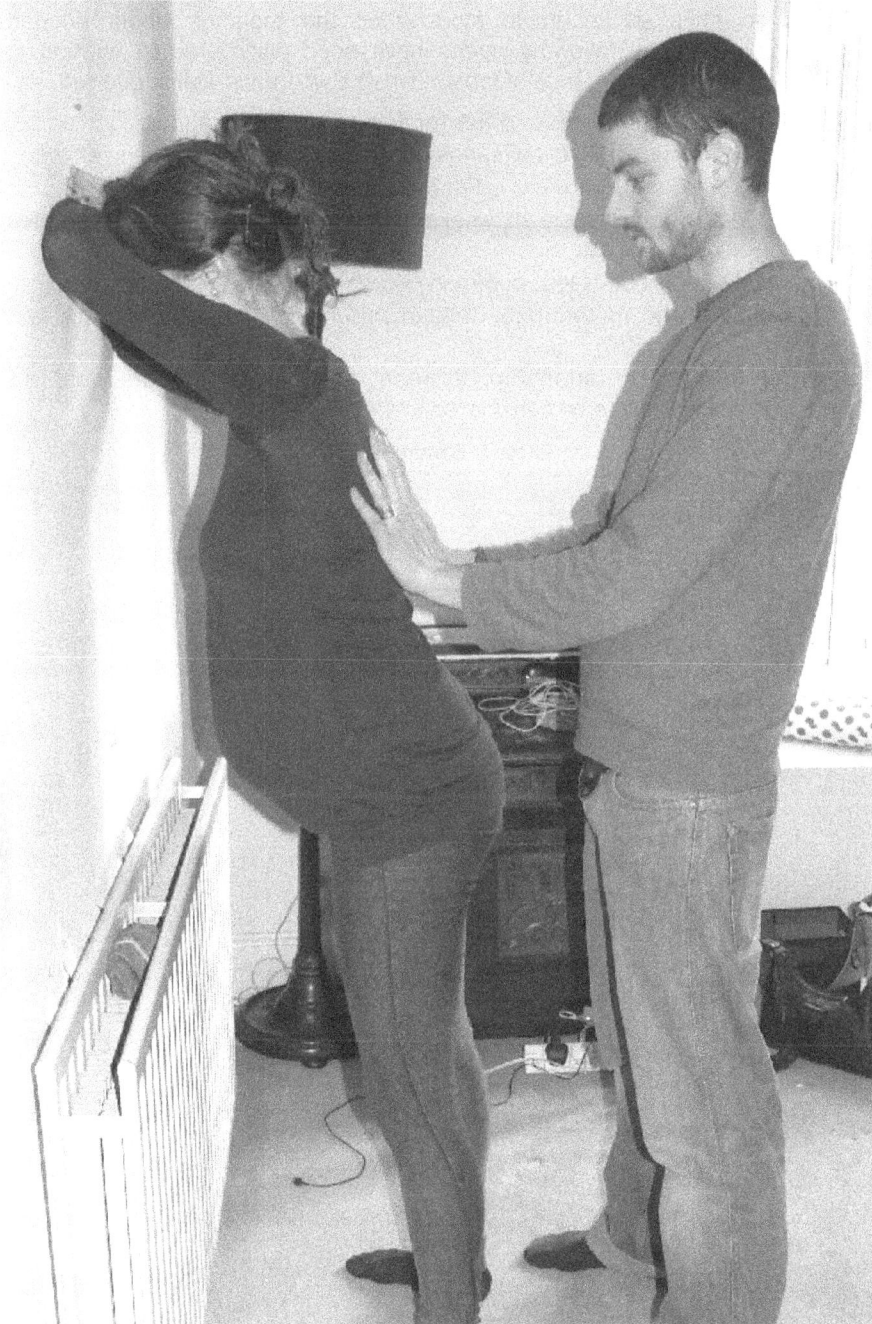

Help or hindrance? For some couples, labour can be a profound, shared experience. What is the situation in your own personal relationship? Can your partner help you?

Even scientific studies have focused on the topic of labour support (Hodnett, 2001). The following points have been discovered in relation to labour pain and the experience of labour, when a woman is well supported:

- Fewer requests are made for drugs for pain relief during labour
- Women report higher levels of satisfaction about their own birthing efforts
- The process of empowerment is felt more clearly
- Breastfeeding usually lasts six weeks longer than when women haven't felt supported during labour
- Postnatal depression is less common
- Difficulties in the mother-baby relationship (and with childcare) are less common
- The professional relationship between the midwife and the woman's partner is less likely to be considered unsatisfactory

Photo © Sandro Pintus

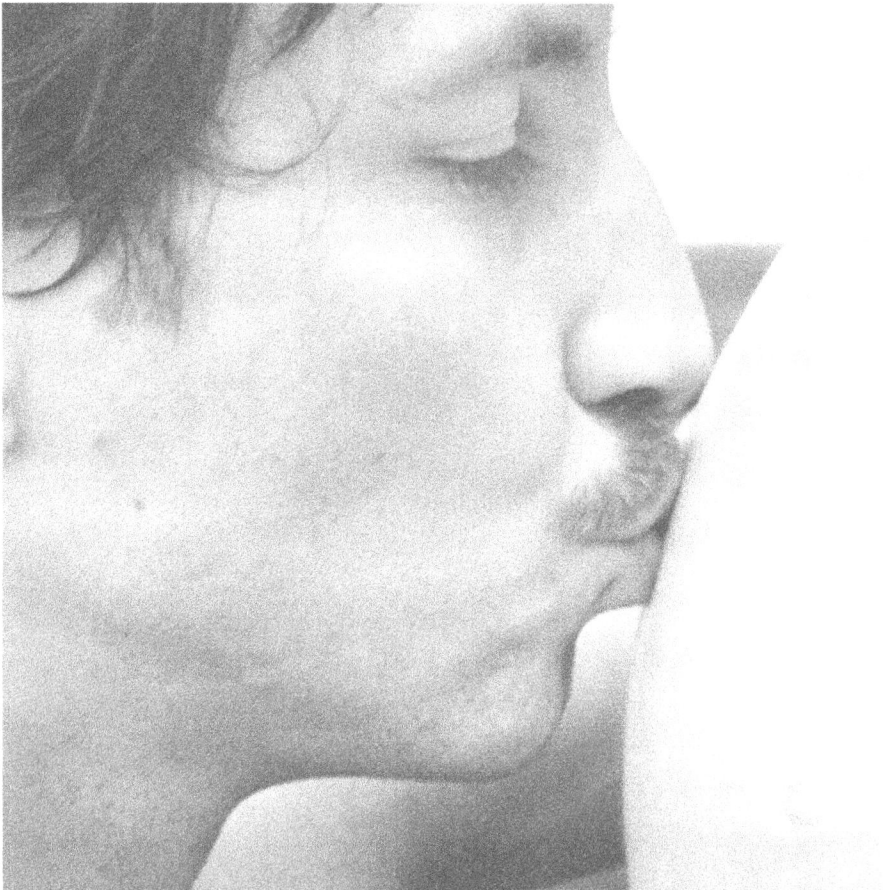

What is your partner's role in the context of labour pain, in your view?

Your partner's role in the context of labour pain

Generally speaking, it is very difficult for a man to impotently watch his life partner experience pain. He lacks the biological qualifications and in Western society he also lacks all the cultural and spiritual requirements necessary to understand, accept and participate in this kind of life experience. A man who decides to be with his partner when she gives birth—something which is today seen as more of a duty than a free choice—must be ready to step from a male realm of experience into a female realm of experience; in other words, he needs to be prepared to step into completely uncharted territory. This is the unknown terrain of subconscious feelings, impulses and instincts, which relate to the element of water, which is a quintessentially feminine area. (See Chapter 6 for more on this.)

In some ancient cultures, there were rituals to help men step into the female territory of birth because doing so was seen as a threat to man's masculinity

In former times and in ancient cultures a father-to-be was helped to step into female territory through social rituals, because moving into this female realm was seen as a threat to a man's masculinity. He therefore had to somehow 'transform' himself into a woman by putting on women's clothes or sharing daily duties and mealtimes with women. This was taken to the point where he sometimes even had to take the pain of birth on to himself and (as if in the woman's place) writhe around and groan in pain. By showing empathy and 'sharing' the experience, he was thought to be protecting his woman from negative influences.

After the birth the new father was required to carry out rituals of courage and force so as to reinstate his manhood and win back his personal and social status as a man. This ritualistic behaviour was an expression of the fears of both the man and the woman in facing the birth experience and this helped to preserve their sense of integrity as individuals and a couple.

Nowadays, only the fears remain... Many women are afraid of freely expressing their instinctual and hidden feelings in front of their partners. After all, they are afraid that they will no longer seem desirable afterwards. At the same time, many men may fear that they will become impotent when they see their partners giving birth and when they share in that experience. And in fact, I have heard that many couples separate in the three years after having a child.

What is useful from all this in our contemporary culture? We need to consider what it might mean today for a man to 'put on womanly clothes' during childbirth, by giving himself up to this (to him) foreign feminine polarity. We need to consider how he can put his 'manly clothes' back on after the birth and turn back to his own masculine polarity. Since we have no social rituals to facilitate this process we need to search out new models of behaviour.

If your birth takes place in a conventional maternity unit with a considerable amount of hi-tech intervention, i.e. in a scenario which is essentially created from masculine norms, the man usually remains a simple observer and sometimes even feels like he is in competition with the medical staff. The more intensive labour pain becomes and the more you express this, the more lost he would feel. He might sense an urgent need to do something. Then, he would run off in search of help, demand that something be done—and while he behaved like this he would remain within the masculine realms of behaviour. He would become more and more anxious and would be extremely tense and inhibited by the technical equipment around him. If he behaved in this way he would disturb your concentration and/or become incapable of really being 'present' for you or communicating with you. The atmosphere of labour would therefore dramatically determine the role he played.

If, on the other hand, the atmosphere in the labour room were to become intimate (which could happen if it's a private room, with little visible technology around, dimmed lighting, a known environment and a comfortable 'lived-in' atmosphere), your partner would more easily be able to find himself a role as a loving and supportive partner. He would then feel able to take on a more feminine role, to find his intuition, to express himself in an appropriate way, according to female norms. He would activate his deep (male) sense of protection for mother and child and for the environment around you both. He would be able to support you as you experience each contraction and offer you relief. He would share with you the stress of each contraction and lovingly relate to you in the breaks between contractions, helping you to relax. Body-to-body contact with you would even allow him to produce birth hormones.

There is a phase during labour and birth (at 7cm-9cm dilation) when it is difficult for anybody to support a labouring woman. The pain is severe, it is usually being expressed without inhibition and with deeply felt emotion. You are likely to find yourself in a situation of maximal opening and you would be expressing your deepest feelings; you might also be completely exhausted and at the end of your tether. (This time is generally called 'transition'.) This is the moment of transformation, of capitulation, of giving up, of fear, of symbolic death of the old 'I' and simultaneously it is the moment of strengthening, when you would be on the point of activating your hitherto unknown inner resources. In actual fact, this process would be greatly facilitated by endorphins and the intense expression of pain would not seem to correspond to the intensity of what you feel. (I have confirmed this many times by speaking to women about their experience after the birth and I can also confirm it from first-hand experience.) You would be in trance.

At this point it is essential that neither your care providers nor your partner disturb this transitional phase. Instead, using encouraging words, in response to cries for help from you—probably claiming that you can't go on—it will be helpful if both your partner and your care providers remember that this is the crucial point in the birthing process and that you will soon regain your strength and feel joyful.

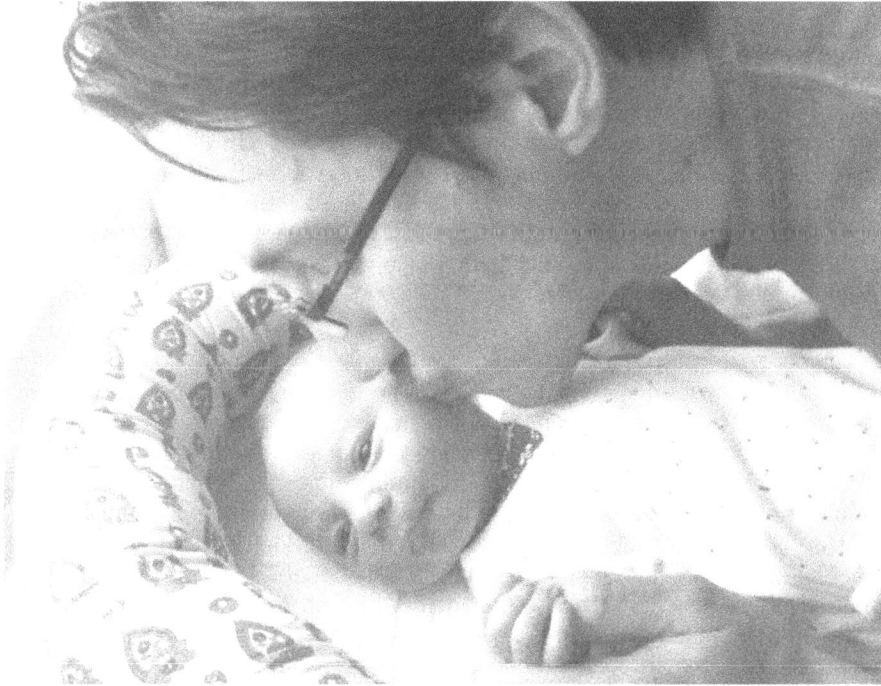

Birth might also be a very intense and emotional experience for your partner

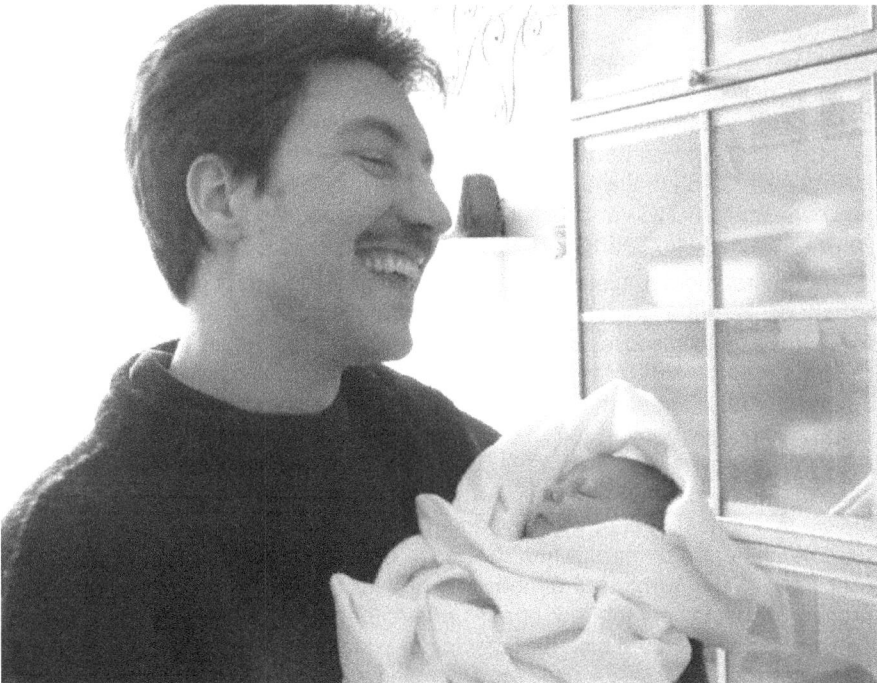

The best way for a man to support you during this phase is to just *be there.* He needs to be open and receptive (i.e. he needs to use feminine qualities) and be totally emotionally available to you. (At that moment you will be encountering your own openness and receptivity.) The sense of 'giving yourself up' you will be experiencing is comparable to the process which takes places during sex. The fear that you may have of 'losing yourself' can be shared with your partner and you can overcome it together, so that you have a sense of complete abandon. If your partner is present to you as a sexual and emotional partner he can support the process by which you are opening up to your baby. After all, as your sexual partner, your man should know how to help you give yourself up completely.

If your partner is unable to support you in this way, it is possible that in this special moment during transition of passivity and fear that your partner will become overwhelmed by feelings of helplessness and despair. If he deals with the feelings in a masculine way, he will feel an urgent need for help and he is likely to insist that care providers intervene in some way. If this happens, or if your partner feels that this phase of labour is unendurable, it is better for him to stand back for a while until you have passed through this phase and start pushing. However, perhaps your midwife will be able to help your partner through this time. Perhaps she can help you both to express your feelings, using her sensitivity, skills and experience—so that you and your partner can continue to move through labour—and perhaps she will effectively end up offering you both support.

If your partner really participates in the birth, he will even participate biologically to a certain extent. He will even rhythmically produce adrenaline when he shares the tension of contractions with you and he will produce endorphins when he relaxes with you in the breaks between each contraction. In this way, labour and birth can be a deeply satisfying experience for him too, and that will help him to bond with his new baby. If at the moment of his baby's birth he is emotionally open and has early skin-to-skin contact with your newborn baby, he will also produce a certain amount of prolactin, along with you . This will trigger caring and tender behaviour.[00]

In the first moments after you have given birth this could mean your partner experiences a kind of identity crisis. (After this kind of experience it is difficult for a man to rediscover male polarity and the feeling of masculinity and redefine it in the light of this experience. The process can be very interesting.) You will therefore need to be very tolerant if your partner pulls back from taking care of your new baby, given that this process is taking place. For you both to retain a healthy relationship after such a profound experience, it is absolutely essential that both you and your partner reorientate yourselves to your proper individual gender polarity. This does not mean giving up a feeling of togetherness or sharing but just that each one of you will need to re-establish your individuality within the dimensions of your relationship. You can help this process by being very tolerant of any unusual behaviour when you are with your partner and you should also be forgiving of yourself, if you behave strangely at any time!

In conclusion, for the male partner labour pain can create stress, anxiety or fear. On the other hand, the experience of supporting you in labour and birth may provide an opportunity for a profound, shared experience, which can help your partner to find his feminine side. A shared labour can also be a catalyst in terms of helping both you and your partner to find your identities and also to develop a sense of identity as a couple. If your partner shares your labour, this may also help him to develop an instinctual sense of protection and responsibility.

The nature of support which is effective

Whoever the birth attendant is—whether it is your partner, your mother or a good friend, it has long been recognised that emotional support is a definitive factor both in your ability to cope with pain and in the context of effecting positive suggestion. Not only have ordinary people accepted this for millennia, but the importance of emotional support in helping you deal with pain and the usefulness of positive suggestion has even been recognised by obstetricians and researchers. Chertok and Langen and Dick-Read were some of the first care providers to accept this. Bonica expressed the view as early as 1977 that interpersonal relationships should be built into a strategy for relieving psychological pain from pregnancy onwards (Bonica, 1977).

You definitely need emotional support if you are going to cope effectively with any pain during labour and birth

Personally, when support is professional, I say it constitutes an 'empathetic relationship'. Suggestion functions mainly on the affective-motivational dimension so it operates on the limbic system. It can be achieved when feelings are shared with good rapport.

In this respect, it is important to have a setup which allows continuous care. The need for this kind of continuous care, for which midwives are the most professionally suited, has been confirmed by numerous studies (for example, that conducted by the World Health Organization in 1996 (WHO, 1996)). The 'support' which needs to take place within this system of continuous care includes...

- **empathetic support**—which means your midwife needs to be a good listener and be accepting of you
- **emotional support**—which means means your midwife needs to use encouragement and reassurance, and be continuously available to you
- **informational support**—which means your midwife needs to provide you with comprehensive information and freedom of choice
- **physical support**—which means your midwife needs to support your body, administering massage, applying compresses (during labour) and offering you food and drink
- **protective support**—which means your midwife needs to recognise and validate your wishes and needs, and deal with them in a way which is suitably respectful, while creating a protected, private environment in which your labour can run its natural course

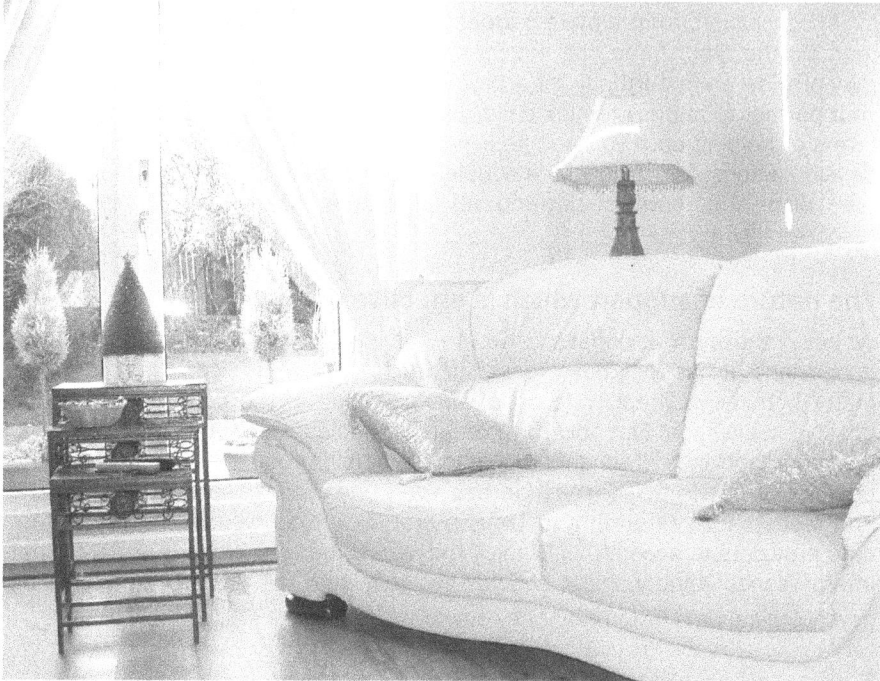

The role of the environment in birth

The constant, dynamic effect of your environment on you and your physiology and psychology is a significant part of your life. We can never consider human beings separately from their environment and it is possible that people behave differently in different environments. Both psychologists and architects focus on 'environmental psychology' and this branch of science researches the psychological and physical changes in people which are caused by the environment in which they find themselves.

Michel Odent explains this effect by referring to neurophysiological mechanisms between your neocortex (your conscious mind) and your archaic brain (your subconscious) (Odent, 1999). Stimuli from the environment, which activate your neocortex (e.g. light, noise, loud voices, calls to reason, actions) stimulate your sympathetic nervous system and inhibit the functioning of your archaic brain. By contrast, the influences from outside which activate your archaic brain (e.g. darkness, intimacy, soft voices, quiet, lack of disturbance and no movement from outside) stimulate your parasympathetic nervous system and inhibit your neocortex. This pattern is comparable to the night-day pattern: during daytime wakefulness, attentiveness and action predominate, rather than sleep, dreams and the activity of the internal organs. When one state predominates, the other, contrasting state becomes inhibited. And precisely this pattern of change is decisive when it comes to health.

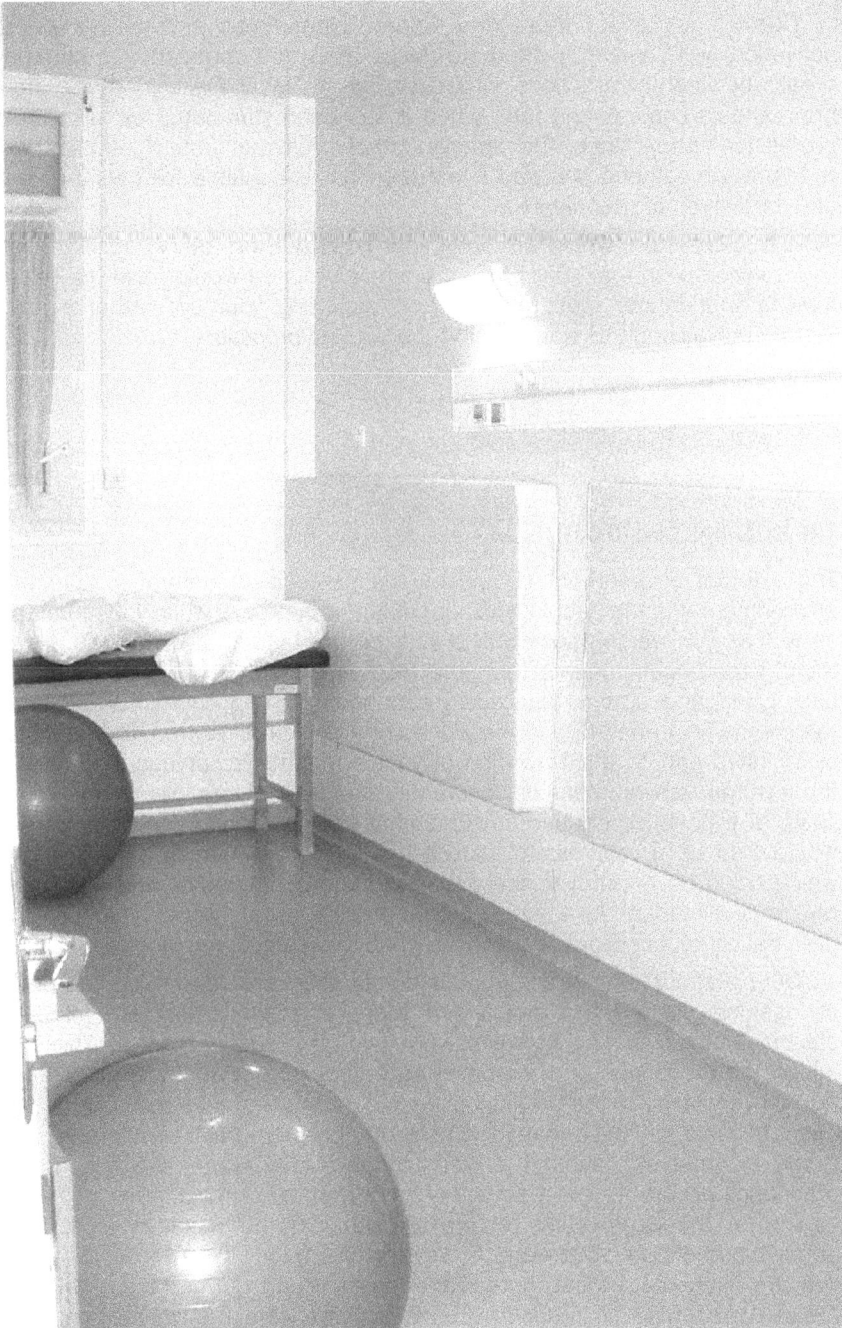

This page and overleaf: *Both the décor and people's behaviour will affect the atmosphere in the room where you are labouring and giving birth*

During your labour these two states (sympathetic and parasympathetic activation) will constantly alternate (since there are contractions, followed by breaks between contractions). However, eventually, the activity of the archaic brain should come to the fore, when it has been stimulated by pain and the production of hormones. The parasympathetic nervous system will then prevail over the sympathetic one and it will then be responsible for opening you up and for dilation of your cervix.

It is this system which will bring your baby out into the world. Stimulating your neocortex so that your archaic brain is inhibited would have the effect of making your labour more difficult and of letting your sympathetic nervous system prevail and this would inhibit the birthing process.

If your neocortex is stimulated, this would inhibit your archaic brain and make your labour more difficult

THE EXTERNAL ENVIRONMENT

The external environment comprises the perceivable natural (or unnatural) environment and the people which inhabit it, around you while you're in labour, as well as your family, society and your birth attendants. Viewed as a whole, these various components form the 'ecosystem' in which you live and your baby grows and is born. Your ecosystem has an effect on your physiology, on the mechanism whereby your neocortex or archaic brains are either stimulated or inhibited and on the activation of your sympathetic nervous system. When the external environment is constantly stimulating your neocortex, you are likely to experience chronic stress during your pregnancy and labour. There would also be a progressive increase in the production of catecholamines, which could be harmful to the progress of your pregnancy and your unborn baby's development. As a result, your endocrine system would be inhibited and prenatal contact between you and your baby would become more difficult.

During labour, effacement and dilation of your cervix and the entire process of opening up will be impeded if there is chronic distress. Instead of catecholamines coming in waves, you would produce cortisol. This would inhibit the production of endorphins and other birth hormones, so you would remain very tense in the breaks between contractions. As a result, your labour might become difficult and involve considerably more pain. On the other hand, if the external environment is very calming and without stimulation, your pregnancy will proceed very smoothly, both from a hormonal point of view and also from the perspective of fetal growth. On the negative side, if your parasympathetic nervous system prevails and there is a lack of stimulation, you are likely to become increasingly passive and during labour this might mean there would be reduced uterine activity, with passive dilation and no force, to such an extent that your baby would be unable to be born.

If you are not stimulated, you will become passive

Subliminal messages sent to you may include gestures and subtle changes in people's behaviour

All kinds of subliminal messages are sent to you from the external environment during your pregnancy and while you're in labour. These may include gestures (and other body language), comments from birth attendants, the décor of the room, and subtle changes in interpersonal behaviour between the people in the room. These all reach your archaic brain and once they are there, they either increase the electrical charge in your central brain structures, or reduce it, depending on what type of message is conveyed. You can be influenced much more easily than women who are not pregnant. As a result, your susceptibility to these subliminal messages from your immediate environment increases. Often, empathetic behaviour, appropriate communication or even a simple change in your environment (to do with light, temperature, air, music, etc.) can reduce your stress levels, change the atmosphere of the room and therefore positively influence the course of your labour and your perception of pain.

Even a simple change in the environment may influence the course of your labour and your perception of pain

Photo © Colin Smith

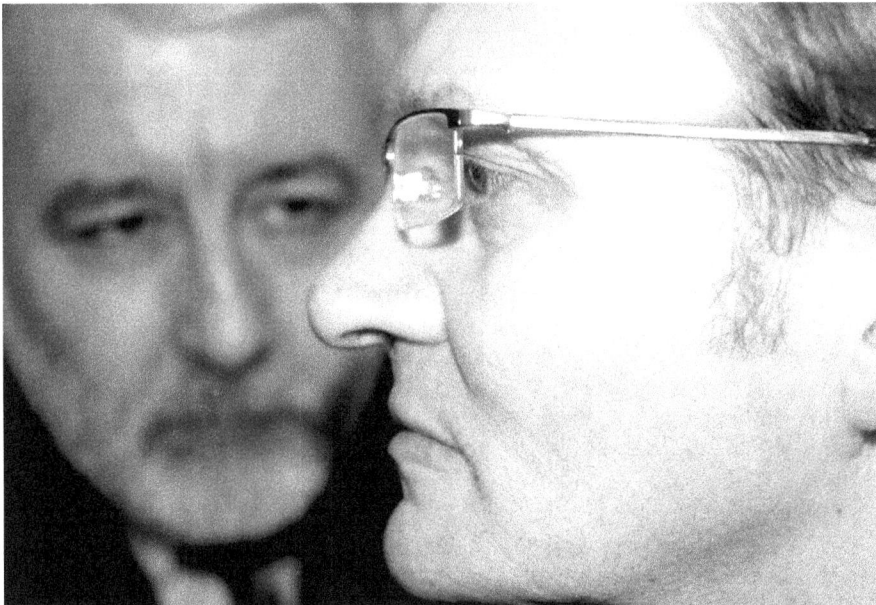

The body language of people around you will reach your archaic brain and either increase the electrical charge in the central brain structures, or reduce it

THE INTERNAL ENVIRONMENT

The internal environment comprises all emotional factors: personal experiences and hearsay, cultural conditioning and social values. If your internal environment is already heavily overburdened with subconscious emotional baggage, this will raise a central alarm as far as increasing stimuli are concerned and block the activation of the inhibiting, pain-lowering mechanism. The more problems are hidden in your subconscious, the bigger the electrical charge. Even this alone can cause you chronic stress, with similar physiological consequences to when stress is caused as a result of the external environment. In the case of stress caused by your internal environment it is just much harder to find out about the stress stimuli, and it's necessary to do this if you are to deal with them. Factors in your external environment can aggravate this problem even more, since they can remind you of internalised negative experiences... even without you realising this consciously, or without your care team understanding.

In these situations there are various things you can do to help yourself, either during your pregnancy or even while you're in labour:

- Join an antenatal class which will allow you to talk about your experiences. If your discussion is facilitated by a good course leader, an exchange of experiences and impressions can be extremely liberating. As I have already suggested, fears become smaller when people name them and talk about what happened. When you do this, you will also extend your repertoire of strategies for coping with your fears. Expressing fears and suffering will allow you to release tensions from the central structures of your brain.
- Positively condition yourself using deep relaxation exercises and visualisation. Using deep relaxation techniques and visualisation can help you bring your deep-seated worries to the surface of your mind. This can help activate inhibitive reactions on the descending pathways.

There are some other things you can do to substantially reduce the impact of other negative factors which might influence the amount of pain you are likely to experience during your labour:

- Ensure you arrange to give birth in a comfortable place, with known people, where you will be warmly welcomed on arrival, and where you will feel safe.
- Find care providers who you know will provide a supportive, trusting environment, and who will allos you to express yourself exactly as you want.
- Relax in the breaks between contractions. As I've already explained, this will support the production of endorphins and the underlying physiological rhythm of your contractions.
- Remember the reasons for the choices you have made for your own labour and help yourself to cope by moving around freely, as you wish. Also, draw support from the people around you.
- During your labour, if anybody around you is browbeating, frightening or intimidating you, or if you feel they might prevent you from expressing yourself totally freely... ask them to leave, and insist that they do so.

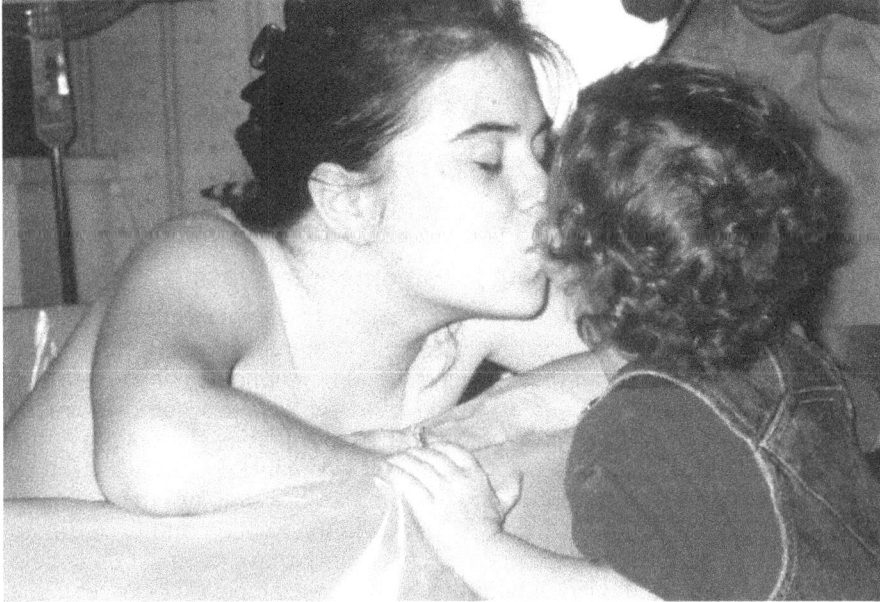

Other people close to you—not just the midwife—might be able to offer you support, depending on the nature of their relationship with you

- Do everything you can to make sure your neocortex is not stimulated in any way, i.e. use dim lighting, make sure the atmosphere around you is calm and explain to people in advance that you must not be disturbed with any questions or instructions.
- Finally, consider using warm water. This can reduce your levels of adrenaline and therefore reduce the level of pain you experience. However, note that it can also reduce your strength and inhibit your fetus ejection reflex.

The importance of a balanced view

In spite of everything, there may be situations in which you cannot cope and nobody can do anything to help you. This may happen if you haven't had the opportunity to meet any other pregnant women before you go into labour, if you don't know your midwife or if you get to the hospital so late that—for administrative reasons—you have no opportunity to build an empathetic relationship with your caregivers. In these cases medical pain relief can have an important therapeutic effect, so it should always be available to you. The essential thing is that you continue to try to work through any discomfort you experience and that you explore ways of making yourself feel better. Your caregivers may well be able to help you in this respect.

CHAPTER 6:

Labour pain as a topic
of study and exploration

Your objectives when looking for an antenatal class

In order to explore the topic of labour pain and methods you can use for dealing with it, you may well consider joining an antenatal class. Various types of classes are available, but they vary considerably in approach and in terms of content. Some classes are geared to the needs of women who have already decided precisely how they want to give birth. (For example, classes run at the Active Birth Centre in London are designed for women who already know they want to have an *active* birth, not one involving an epidural, or other forms of drug-based pain relief.) These women just need information and exercises to help them get the birth they want. Other classes may have been set up to help the women decide what kind of birth they want (for example NCT classes). Still other classes may have been set up to *prepare* women for birth in a particular institution (e.g. hospital-based classes, which are run by midwives who work on a large maternity ward). Obviously, the methods and content of any classes will be affected by where they are due to take place, by the preconceived ideas of the teacher and by requests from other women registered for the classes.

In antenatal classes which aim to prepare you for an active birth, you shouldn't be taught any 'recipe for success', involving breathing or other techniques. The work you do in the classes should focus on only one objective: to put you in touch with yourself and your instinctual knowledge, i.e. with your body's own knowledge of how to give birth. And as far as the topic of pain management is concerned, antenatal classes should help you to free your 'pain pathways' and enable you to function in a completely physiological way.

Changing the value or meaning of pain for you

In order to address the issue of pain, you will need to focus on the cognitive-evaluating dimension of pain. We have already seen how cultural factors might give pain a negative meaning in your mind. You might see it as unnecessary suffering, punishment, loss of control, being delivered up to negative forces, the price of having a child, a danger to your own integrity and health, dangerous also for your child, etc. If you evaluate pain negatively in this way, this will influence your affective-motivational system of pain perception, so that you meet pain with reactions of flight and retreat. At the same time, these evaluations would affect the sensory-perceptive dimension and would reduce your pain threshold. However, if in the classes you discuss cultural aspects of labour pain and its function and possible ways of experiencing it, you can also change its value on a cognitive level. Reactions to sensations then change: you will perceive pain positively, as strength, as rhythm, as a wave, as exertion, as 'good pain' or similar, and you may even perceive it as being almost pleasant.

There is then no avoidance response, involving displeasure, flight and withdrawal. The affective-motivational system will send reassuring messages to your reticular system, which will then send inhibitive, downscaling stimuli to the posterior horns of your spinal cord, which will further reduce your perception of pain (on the sensory-perceptive level). In this way, endorphins will be produced and your feeling of fulfilment will be strengthened.

For you, changing pain in this way is invaluable... You will become aware of a resource and a capability within your own body. This resource will become part of your biological competence and a little simple work on a cognitive level will change the chemistry of your body and some of its most important neurophysiological functions.

Practical approaches to learning about pain management

In your antenatal class or with a group of trusted friends, try the following...

1: Share your experience and perceptions

Talk about your experiences of pain and consider its specific cultural background in each case. You can begin to explore where your views on pain come from by considering a few simple questions:

- What do I think of pain?
- How do I feel when I think of pain?
- What has pain meant to me in other situations in my life?
- What do I imagine labour pain to be like?

Get views from as many people as possible. When you're working in a small group facilitate the process of exploration using various methods, including brainstorming, group work and anonymous messages on slips of paper. Either your class teacher or a nominated facilitator in an informal group, should bring the various comments together in periodic summaries.

Use other techniques too to bring out your own and other participants' experiences and views... For example, you could ask your teacher to do a guided visualisation of pain memories in different phases of life (childhood, adolescence, adulthood). Try the following (or similar) wording...

- Think back to any physical or spiritual pain you have experienced. How did it feel? How strong was the pain? What was your first reaction to it?
- What or who helped you deal with the pain? What role did your body play and what role did your mind play?
- Which feelings did you experience most strongly when you'd overcome the pain?
- How was pain different during different phases of your life? What was the same?
- What kind of support would have helped you deal with the pain more successfully?
- What resources could you use in the face of pain? Do you remember how you coped ,or could you imagine how you might cope?

This might then lead to a sharing of successful 'pain tools'. You can do this in the following way. On a whiteboard or flipchart one person in the group should write down the various strategies you and other participants suggest for dealing with pain, which you all think might be helpful. You are likely to find that a long list of strategies will quickly appear. It's striking how many resources we have within ourselves for dealing with pain, without needing to request medical help. Here are some of the strategies previous groups of mine have come up with...

'PAIN TOOLS' WHICH HAVE BEEN FOUND TO BE USEFUL

- Distract yourself—think of something pleasant, not of the pain itself.
- Think about when the pain will be over; hope and wait for that time.
- Breathe the pain 'out'; blow it out; breathe consciously and relax; breathe deeply.
- Breathe *into* the pain and mindfully sink into it.
- Get to the point where you can more consciously experience the pain... Where is it exactly? How 'big' is it?
- Simply be aware; concentrate on your surroundings; smooth the pain away.
- Concentrate on the pain, so that it can dissolve.
- Know that you are stronger than the pain—and therefore push the pain into a corner.
- Be aware that the pain is of limited duration; know its cause and concentrate on that fact.
- Concentrate on the positive aspects of the experience which accompany the pain.
- Talk the pain 'down' (e.g. "It could be much worse!") so as to come to terms with it.
- Understand the reason for the pain; accept it; give into it; let it come so that it can then go again (in a tension-release cycle).
- Imagine a light at the end of a tunnel ("Sometime soon, the pain will be gone").
- Mindfully and gently allow yourself to become engulfed in the pain... Cats roll around in pain!.
- Visualise a distant landscape, and see the pain fade away into the distance.
- Mindfully isolate the painful part of the body and relax the painfree parts of the body.
- Listen to beautiful words; imagine beautiful words yourself (spoken in a pleasant voice).
- See the pain as part of yourself. Pain means encountering your own ego.
- Concentrate on a point in the distance so as to mentally distance yourself from the pain.
- Don't move, so that you don't alter the pain (i.e. maintain a protective posture which minimises the pain).

- Alternatively, move around so as to change the pain.
- Make some rhythmic movements—for example sway, bounce, shake, dance, loosen up, run round in circles.
- Sleep, rest, meditate.
- Have a warm bath (imagining that the pain is dividing itself up, going out of the body, or being dissolved).
- Use hot water bottles and/or hot compresses.
- Use cold things; stay in a cold place.
- Use aromatherapy or music.
- Don't let yourself be overcome by the pain; instead let yourself jump the wave of pain at just the right moment.
- Affirm the pain; give it permission to exist—note this is also important for other people in the birth space.
- Get wrapped up in a cosy blanket; find a sheltered hollow where it's possible to stay focused inward; don't feel or be alone.
- Hole up somewhere; wrap up warm; stay alone and undisturbed; don't allow any distractions.
- Vocalise (i.e. moan and groan); sigh; scream; howl; sob; sing; intone sounds; rant and rave.
- Be comforted and consoled; get taken care of; be reassured ("You can do it!").
- Have your hand held and thereby feel someone else's strength and sense of safety.
- Have someone lay their hands on you or lay your own hands on painful areas.
- Hand the pain over to someone else; share it.
- Concentrate on contrasting sensations.
- Apply firm pressure to the painful spot; rub it; massage any painful areas.
- Apply firm pressure to another part of the body so as to produce 'counter-pain' as a distraction.
- Get some bodily contact; be taken up into someone else's arms; be stroked; be supported.
- Perform rituals (repeat religious words, breathe rhythmically); be supported by your own mother.
- Imagine the pain before it happens.
- Have your feet massaged; mindfully let the pain flow into the earth, out through your feet.
- Close your eyes; stay in the dark; have dim lighting; go to sleep; drift away into another state of consciousness.
- Drink some hot tea; have some food; eat chocolate.
- Go for a walk in the countryside; breathe in fresh air; feel the earth underneath your feet.
- Be open to the needs of your body; let yourself go deep within; tune into your body.

2: Learn about the physiology of pain

Of course it is neither possible nor meaningful to talk about the type of pain different women have and it is not possible to anticipate the experience you will have because it's bound to be very individual for you. Nevertheless, you can continue to learn about the physiological mechanisms of pain, as well as its protective and awareness-raising functions. As a result, you will be able to see a positive meaning in labour pain; you will be able to recognise its role in helping you develop and grow; and then you will be able to make an active, informed choice about how you deal with it.

So as to really deeply motivate yourself to actively come to grips with labour pain, you need to recognise your own, deep needs, which can be fulfilled through the experience of pain. A few of the positive images which might help you to do this might be: seeing pain as a challenge, as a test of strength and a way of using your deep resources; as a personal test; as a source of knowledge; as the experience of something mysterious; as a signpost; as a way of experiencing separation from your baby within you; as a protective mechanism; as a means of regaining your independence...

3: Reflect on what you're learning and feeling

After these discussions it's important to continue exploring your feelings as a group. Some questions which might help you to reflect and which might open up the discussion could be as follows:

- What's my view of labour sensations and pain now?
- Have any of the things that have been said been particularly meaningful to me?
- Is there anything I haven't understood?
- Did I particularly like some of the things that were said?
- Is there anything I've disagreed with?
- Is one specific aspect of labour pain particularly easy for me to imagine?
- What do I still feel I need in order to deal with any pain I might experience?

4: Consider your freedom and choice in childbirth

Most women in Western societies have a particular view of birth, which lies somewhere between the technological model and a completely natural birth. They see birth in hospitals as a safe option and regard some routine procedures as being necessary or bearable, although they would like to be informed about them, and they want to decide for themselves which procedures are carried out, or at least they want to *participate* in the decision-making which takes place amongst caregivers. Basically, they accept the technological model or at least don't question it to any great extent, partly because it's the model on which society and the working world are both based. All these women ask is to actively participate within this system, so as to subtly alter it. Their sense of satisfaction and the 'success' (or otherwise) of their own birthing experience is less dependent on how the birth itself went as on how well the birth matched their particular set of values and expectations and how much control and decision-making power they had.

You may feel free if you have more personal power than caregivers or an institution and can assert this

These women define their own freedom according to the extent to which they have personal power, compared to their caregivers or the institution, and according to the amount of power they are able to assert. Freedom of choice generates its own value system but freedom is not an absolute concept... It is linked to personal perceptions of being able to assert one's needs and knowledge, and make decisions. The sense of freedom any woman has is always linked to the amount of freedom which that particular woman desires, or feels entitled to. Nevertheless, there are basic freedoms, which are so meaningful for human beings that they are mentioned in the constitutions of democratic states. One of these basic freedoms is your right not to have your own body violated, i.e. it is the right to maintain your own body's integrity. This is why you can freely make decisions about any medical intervention which might threaten the integrity of your body. Exceptions are only made in emergency cases and in some countries in the case of compulsory vaccinations. Not being able to move around freely during such an intense event as childbirth, or being forced to adopt positions which are harmful to your health, could be seen to constitute an infringement of your basic human rights.

If you are not sufficiently consulted before an intervention (which might affect either you or your baby), and you are not involved in the decision-making process, this contravenes your legal right to consent. However, it is difficult to avoid the situation where you are insufficiently consulted within a system of routine protocols in a clinic or hospital, for example in an emergency. This is why a discussion of typical procedures and rituals in hospital environments is an essential component of any antenatal classes.

Some of the key questions to get you thinking about this are as follows... Who should decide how much freedom and choice you have during your labour and birth, which is one of the most important and difficult times in your life? Can you determine your care yourself or should it always be determined by a patriarchal and technocratic society, in which women's bodies and therefore also their strength are controlled? To what extent are you aware of this kind of control being exerted over you and to what extent do you accept this control because of the deep feeling of inadequacy you perceive when it comes to your ability to give birth? Moving towards freedom—and even to the amount of freedom which you personally would like to have for yourself—should be your task in any series of discussions or antenatal classes.

If only you would transmute this feeling of inadequacy into a demand for support, of the type you could control yourself, you would be able to safeguard your basic freedom and you would be able to put the system to good use. Instead, you may prefer merely to suffer under it. This transmutation of feeling can be a transitional phase, a gradual but necessary transformation on the way towards freedom in birth, which strengthens your sense of self-worth.

The most important element of classes, in terms of helping you grow towards freedom, is to give you correct and comprehensive information. This should include information about care you might receive during your labour and birth, general physiology, different birthplaces (hospitals, birth centres and home) and the different types of pain relief available (including details about their advantages and disadvantages). In this way, you will work on the cognitive-evaluating dimension of pain.

During antenatal classes you can also draw up a birth plan (or 'care guide'). This simply means putting everything down on paper that is relevant to the care you would like to receive during your labour and birth. In order to do this, you need to be aware of your individual needs. After discussing what these might be, you should write down:

- what you would *fight for*—simply because these details represent what you see as being your basic, inviolable freedoms
- what you would *negotiate*—because these details relate to non-essential needs, which you are happy to compromise on
- what has been *agreed*—in terms of what's on offer and what you have chosen in terms of your birthplace and type of care.

As far as possible, it's good if you can include mostly points which have been agreed upon, because it's necessary to trust the birthing environment during labour and birth. In cases where there is not much agreement on specific points, the choice of birthplace should be thought through again. Where possible, all points on a care guide should be fully discussed with a midwife or consultant beforehand.

When it's ready, a copy of your care guide can be kept with your medical notes and you can also take a copy along to the birth itself. It is important that your midwife and also any other caregivers accept that you have the right to decide what you would fight for and what you are prepared to negotiate. They need to accept that it is not their task to make this decision for you.

Your requests can gradually change the system of care given to labouring women. If midwives hold back on providing information to you and other pregnant women because they are afraid of triggering a 'crisis of confidence', they are preventing you from making choices and are thereby limiting your freedom. At the same time, midwives must not use you as a tool for achieving their own ends and they mustn't burden you with the responsibility of changing a system, which—in the view of some women—seems to be built on mysterious and incomprehensible logic. Since midwives know the system, they should accept responsibility for changing it from within.

What you want for your own labour and birth will be determined by your personal, individual needs. Changes suggested by a midwife should only be proposed for clinical reasons or because the midwife would like to improve the quality of care you receive.

An example of an individual care guide [with blank lines for choices]

During my labour and birth and afterwards, the following points are important to me and I would ask my caregivers to respect them:

During labour...

- I do not want to be prepped in any way.
- I want to be allowed to eat and drink during labour, as I wish.
- For fetal monitoring, I would like the following:

  _____

- I would like to have the freedom to move around as I wish during my entire labour and birth.
- I will deal with any pain I experience using

  _____

- I agree to interventions, where these are considered necessary, only after I have been given a full explanation of the circumstances and have been fully consulted. I do not consent to the following:

  _____
  _____
  _____

During the birth...

- Positions I would like to use for the birth itself might include

  _____

- My birth attendants may/will be

  _____

- I do not want to have any perineal stretching or an episiotomy.

After the birth...

- To facilitate bonding and undisturbed skin-to-skin contact after the birth I would appreciate the following:

  _____
  _____

- I do not want you to administer Vitamin K, antibiotics or anything else to my newborn baby, without asking my consent.
- I would like to have a physiological third stage, if my birth was normal.
- I plan to breastfeed and do not want you to arrange any supplementary feeding.
- I would like to have my baby with me at all times.

THE CONCEPT OF 'INFORMED CHOICE'

In practice this means the following:

- You should be provided with comprehensive information, based on up-to-date research evidence, in a sensitive way, without any browbeating or fear-mongering.
- Clear explanations should be provided about alternatives available, including details of advantages and disadvantages.
- Each intervention should be explained in an unprejudiced, balanced way (with information about positive and negative aspects of each intervention). Explanations should include information on procedures, their rationale, advantages, consequences, side-effects and risks.
- You yourself must be allowed to decide what type and level of risk is acceptable for you.
- A detailed description needs to be provided of any special implications of making a particular choice.
- Your caregiver should make sure that you fully understand what you have been told.
- Sufficient time should be provided for you to think through the physical, psychological and emotional consequences of each of your decisions.
- Decisions which a specialist needs to make in the case of an emergency should be identified in advance. Decisions can be identified as such only in cases where it would not be possible for you and your partner to have the necessary information to make a decision.
- You should be assured of having complete support and respect from your midwives, even in cases where a midwife disagrees with a particular decision you have made.
- Midwives need to understand that you have a well-developed protective instinct when it comes to your unborn baby's welfare. Unless you are a drug addict or suffer from mental illness you will always want to do the best thing possible for your unborn baby.
- Midwives need to understand that you and your baby are an inseparable entity. Accepting this basic principle, your midwife will need to support you in every situation during your pregnant, labour and also postnatally .

All this is extremely important because if you give birth to your baby in the strength of your own ability to make decisions and/or by dint of your own capabilities (supported and free, or in accordance with your own wishes) and if you can hold your baby straight after the birth, you will proudly describe the self-confidence and even ecstasy, which you have gained through this experience.

If you give birth yourself, if you can hold your baby straight away... you will feel confident—ecstatic!

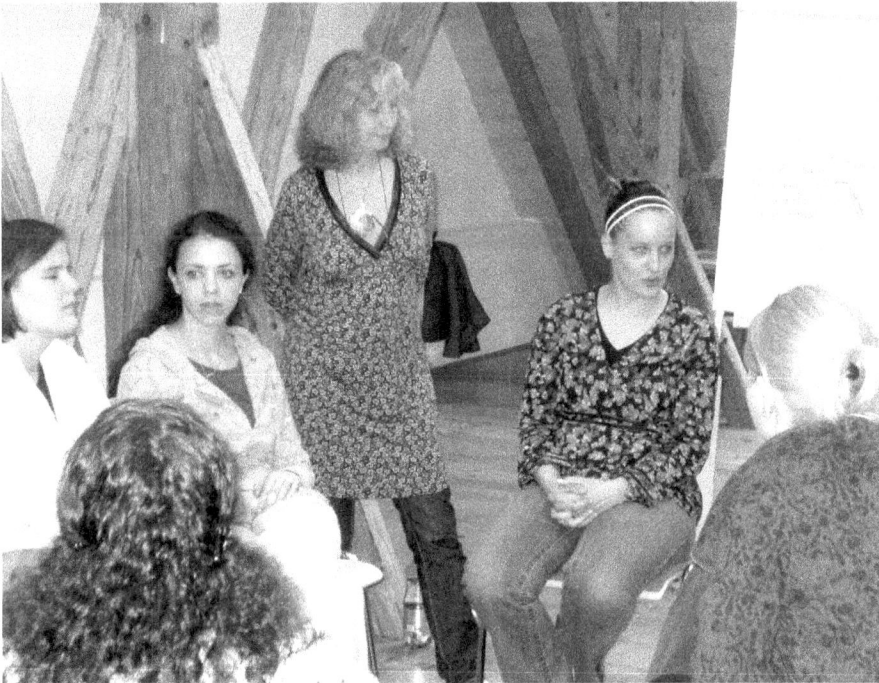

Working in pairs or small groups in an antenatal class, you will be able to consider what's important for you for your own labour and birth

EMPOWERMENT

In the transitional period from the current system of 'demand for care' towards another healthcare system which will involve maintaining health, rather than dealing with illness, you need a new form of empowerment and you need to become stronger. After all, in the current system there is the tendency to see health as a consumer good, while in the new system you, as the client, will assume responsibility for yourself and your health and you will participate in the system which maintains your health.

In the technological model of birth, empowerment means going beyond passive, consumer-oriented, uncritical behaviour (or regressive coping) when faced with technologically-oriented medicine. This is possible when you have factual information about processes which take place during labour and birth (and even during illness) and when you have ways of dealing with those processes. It is also possible when you develop enough inner strength to see through a previously thought-out choice.

If you like the idea of empowerment and an 'empowered' model of birth, you will probably want to have a lot of information which you can process cognitively. During your labour and birth you will want to know precisely which point you're at in your labour, you will want to avoid unnecessary interventions, you will want to participate in all decision-making, even when interventions are considered necessary. This means that—given all your knowledge—you will want to have a certain level of control over your labour and birth. In this kind of case, your sense of satisfaction with your birthing experience will depend less on what actually happens and much more on the extent to which you personally perceive that you have maintained control over the processes of labour and birth. Your sense of satisfaction will also be influenced by how much you feel you were able to exercise your personal power and by the extent to which your expectations were met.

The experience of birth can then be linked to your self-assertiveness and 'empowerment', even in cases where you do not agree with your birth attendants about certain interventions. This is because the way in which interventions are carried out and their timing may be influenced by your own decisions, or at least by your expression of your personal wishes, and if your needs are respected, you may still value your experience positively.

Generally, when empowerment is considered, it is associated with an increase in personal power. This kind of strengthening of power can be achieved when you get to know your midwife better and when you become more in touch with yourself, i.e. when you listen to yourself, recognise your own needs (on the basis of experience), mobilise your resources and thereby activate a healing process, as well as grow self-confidence and self-awareness. All these factors will help you to free yourself from your probable over-dependency on the health care services, they will improve your health and they will also result in a less expensive healthcare system!

During a physiological process such as childbirth it is relatively easy to assert your wishes because pregnancy and birth are natural processes which are usually straightforward. In theory, at least, it should be easy for you to facilitate a good outcome—although, in practice, this positive outcome is only more likely if you have a good idea of your real personal needs and use all the resources you have available to you. It is the task of antenatal classes to allow and facilitate the process of empowerment during pregnancy, so as to ensure that pregnancy is undisturbed and also so as to communicate any necessary information which will lead towards your assertiveness.

However, you need to be aware that there is an important qualitative difference between two types of empowerment: one results from an increase in knowledge (cognitive) and one grows out of your attitude (i.e. it comes from your motivation). In the latter case this empowerment naturally expresses itself through your behaviour. However, every woman starts out at the point where she finds herself, and from then on gradually develops. Every woman brings her baby into the world in a way which corresponds to her way of living and she can only be the person she is on any one specific day. So what kind of woman are you? What are your real motivations and wishes?

If only you could become aware of the enormous strength hidden deep inside you... If you were aware of it, you wouldn't just make changes in the areas of pregnancy and birth, but in the whole of society.

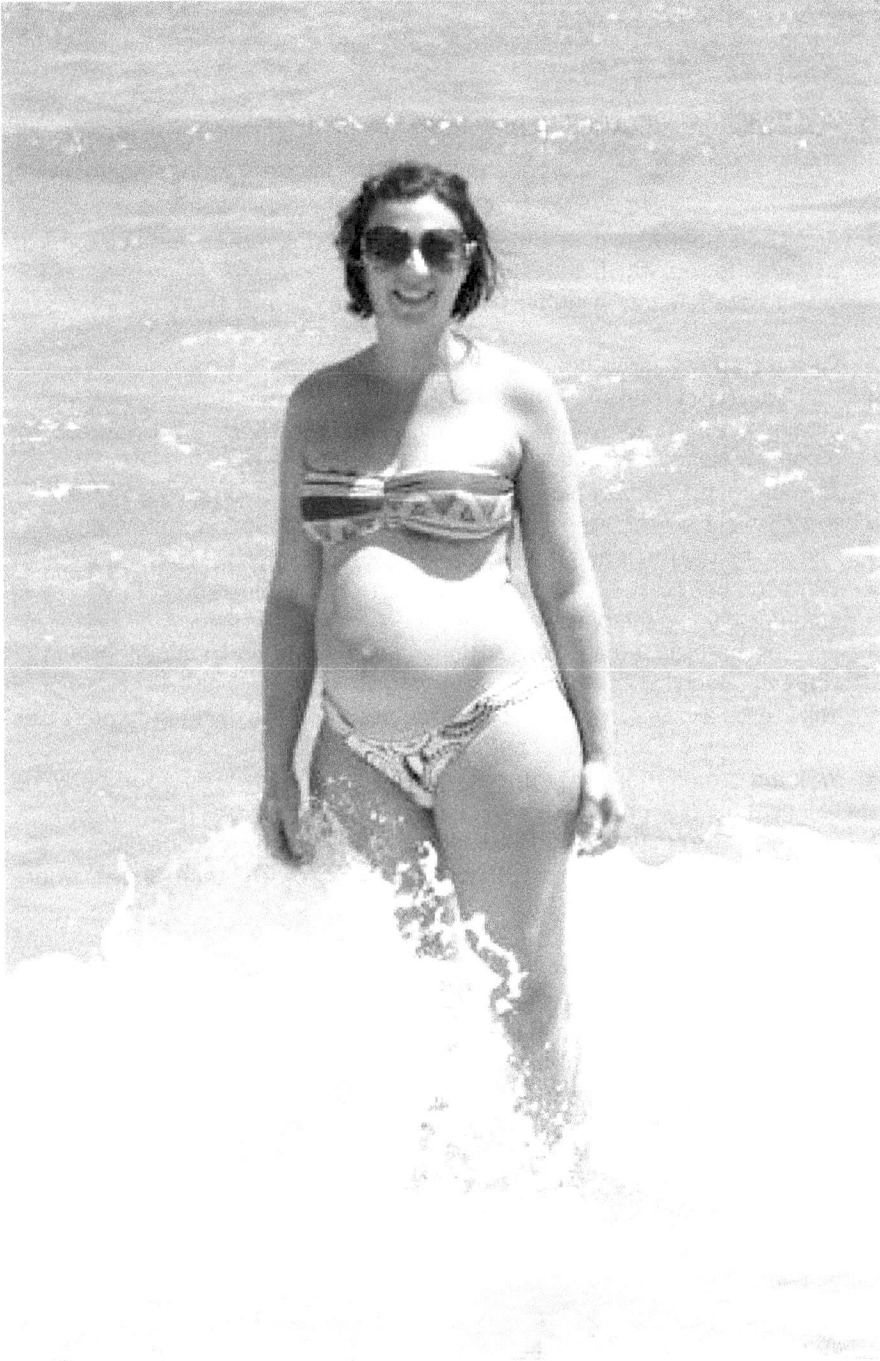

Birth is an elemental force that can strengthen you

If only you were aware of your enormous strength

5: Decide where you want to give birth

You can decide on an appropriate birthplace by considering the following questions...

- Are good healthcare facilities available and good statistical records available to you, which are easy enough to understand?
- Do the staff follow a unified vision of care, or are there variations in approach?
- Do the staff regularly undertake in-service training?
- Can you be certain of having a midwife at your side during your entire labour and birth, as well as other people of your choice? Will you receive emotional support as well as help coping with the pain?
- Are natural methods of pain relief available, as well as drug-based ones?
- Is it possible to get to know the team of midwives during your pregnancy?
- Will you be informed about any routine procedures during your labour?
- Will your personal wishes about the birth be respected while you're in labour, including the ones you've included in your care guide?
- Will you be included in any decision-making which concerns either you or your unborn child?
- Will you be allowed to have the time you need and the rhythm you prefer, as long as there are no signs of pathology?
- Will an atmosphere of intimacy and respect towards your body be safeguarded and protected?
- Will vaginal examinations only carried be out with the your consent?
- Are rooms in labour wards all private rooms or are there areas where several women labour together?
- Will you be able to move around freely at all times and adopt positions which seem helpful to you? Will you be forced to adopt positions which don't suit you?
- Will decisions which you make during your pregnancy (in the weeks running up to the birth) be respected by staff?
- Will you be allowed to give birth to your baby in a way which suits your own philosophy of life? Will you and your new baby have sufficient time to get to know each other thoroughly, in an undisturbed environment in the birthing room itself (e.g. in the delivery suite)—without any separation occurring?
- Will you be offered help in cases where you experience problems postnatally? Will you be supported by a competent advisor?
- Will you be allowed to behave towards your baby in a way which seems good to you?
- Will your rights also be upheld in difficult situations, which require special measures and interventions?

6: Learn specific pain management techniques

You cannot approach this form of learning in an exclusively rational manner. Since it is necessary for you to work with all dimensions of pain it is important to include body work (the experiential dimension) and relaxation exercises (the subconscious and personal dimension).

As we've already seen, your body has many ways of dealing with pain and making it bearable. There are various techniques and approaches on the topic of pain, which you can discuss and practise during antenatal classes. Different midwives running antenatal classes are likely to emphasise different aspects of pain, depending on their own personal interpretation of pain. I would personally encourage you to find an 'elemental' scheme, based on the elements of nature, because this is likely to meet your needs and also take into account the various entry ports of pain. (See 'The Dimensions of Pain' in Chapter 2 for more on this.) This approach echoes the view expressed by Ina May Gaskin in her book *Spiritual Midwifery* (1978). She described pregnant women as 'elemental forces', likening them to gravity, thunderstorms, earthquakes and hurricanes.

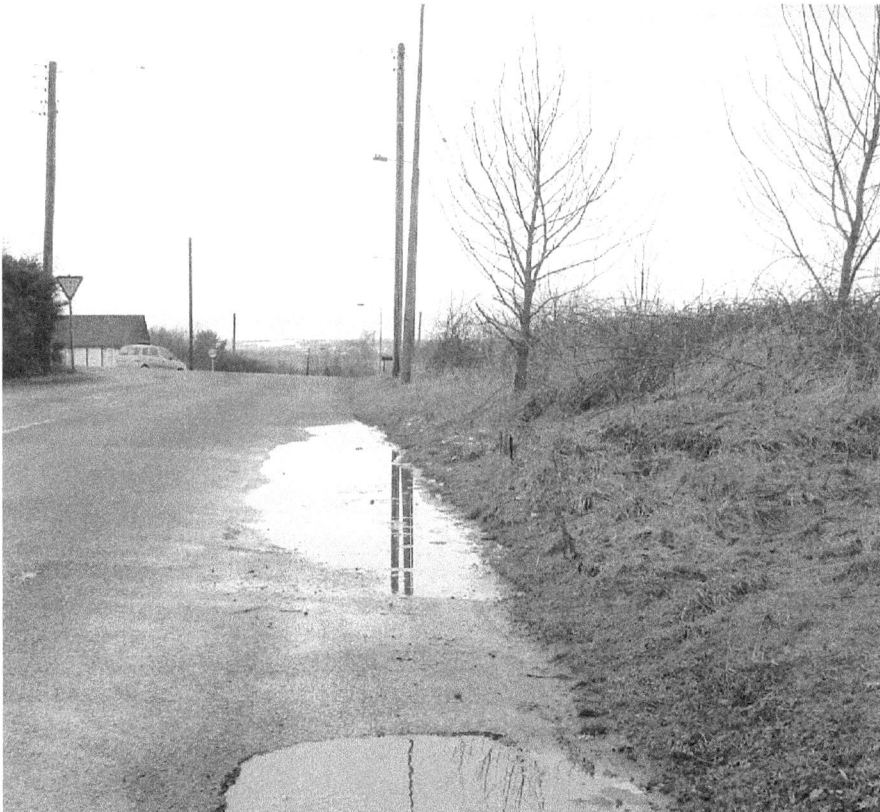

Can you perceive the strength and power within yourself?

7: Work with symbols

During antenatal classes, focusing on the elements will help you to activate your inner resources. I'm talking about four symbolic elements: 'earth', 'water', 'fire' and 'air'. Each has different associations and conveys different images.

- The 'earth' element involves physical contact and stamina
- The 'water' element involves sexuality, self-surrender, opening up and trust
- The 'fire' element involves reactivity, movement, force, capability and decision-making
- The 'air' element involves breathing, singing, rhythm and flexibility

In the rooms where you have your antenatal classes, or where you work in a small group, and even in the rooms in which you labour and give birth, it's possible to integrate pictures and symbols of the four elements, which also leave room for your own internal images and imagination. Here are a few practical examples, to explain how working with the elements can be helpful:

- It's possible the balance of elements in you may be subtly disturbed at the beginning of your pregnancy by the presence of your baby. If this is the case you would feel as if you have been catapulted forcefully into the 'water' element (which is the source of life and the emotions). This means that you would feel ill at ease, you would produce more saliva and you would be susceptible to nausea and morning sickness. If this sounds like you, it could be helpful to work on the 'earth' element (which curtails the production of water and sucks up any residual water) because this might quickly help you to find relief from your symptoms.
- If, during the second trimester of your pregnancy, you feel stressed out, tense, hyperactive and fearful, stimulating the 'water' element may be helpful because this should slow you down and enable you to get in touch with your feelings—and this would help you to make contact with the baby growing within you. (If you are tense, hyperactive and fearful there is also the possibility you might be producing too little amniotic fluid and/or that your baby could be growing too slowly.) As well as helping you to slow down and tune into your baby, working on the 'water' element should also mean that your placenta should start functioning more efficiently. Working on the 'earth' element is likely to help you feel trusting and safe.
- If you are suffering from oedema (water retention) this can be helped when the 'air' element is stimulated. Working on this element brings about movement and promotes good circulation.
- Working on the elements will not only strengthen you, it should also help you to properly nourish your growing baby and it should balance out and harmonise both you and your baby (particularly in terms of your relationship) and it should activate your inner resources. It is work which should usefully prepare you for birth and the pain of labour.
- While you are in labour or giving birth, if you feel that you have no more strength or motivation it's helpful if you work on the 'fire' element. This should make you start producing oxytocin again and it should give you the impulse to push out your baby.

FIRE – THE DYNAMIC-AFFECTIVE LEVEL

Fire is the element of transformation. It burns away the old, brings in the new and introduces light and warmth into the equation. Fire means 'expansion' and its action is centrifugal and dynamic, working from within you and radiating outwards. Fire determines the pattern of pains you will experience, it will give you strength, it will stimulate your sympathetic nervous system and will bring your baby out into the outside world.

Fire is the element of transformation

Completely uninhibited movement has an enormous effect in terms of reducing the pain you will experience. Pain has the enormously helpful function of making you move in such a way that any pressure on your joints and nerves in your pelvis, as well as on your unborn baby's head, is minimised. Moving about freely also means that afferent pain stimuli are reduced.

Free, uninhibited expression of pain is part of the fire element. Freely expressing pain, in a completely uninhibited way, will strengthen your feeling that 'certain things needs to come out' (whirling outwards from within, with a centrifugal force). Movement will also minimise your perception of pain. Means of expressing the 'fire' element include your ability to react and behave actively. In fact, you will become more and more active and expressive, the further along your labour is, i.e. the more active you are, the more 'active' your labour will become. Being active will reduce your pain.

A birth which involves too little 'fire' (pain) proceeds slowly and in a repressed way (i.e. it is hypotonic). A birth with *too much* 'fire', on the other hand, is violent, fast and expulsive (hypertonic). 'Water' (involving feelings and total surrender) and 'earth' (involving a slowing down and pressure) dampen down the 'fire' element (your pain), while 'air' (which involves understanding and the intellect) stokes the fire up and intensifies the pain.

The contrast between contractions ('fire') and the deep relaxation which occurs in the breaks between contractions ('water') is essential if you are to tolerate the pain of labour. This rhythm of change belongs to the 'fire' element. On the other hand, if your labour and birth involves too much 'fire', getting into some water (e.g. in a birthing pool or bath) could have the effect of dramatically reducing the amount of pain you experience.

In order to activate the 'fire' element in your body you will need to ask your midwife or a birth partner to stimulate your eyes (as explained overleaf), your solar plexus and your thighs. Explain in advance to the person who does this that movements to promote the 'fire' element need to be fast and free, that touch needs to be very superficial and stimulating, and that body work will often make you use your voice (i.e. you are likely to vocalise in response).

Have your eyes, solar plexus and thighs stimulated

Sample exercises

A few tools of the 'fire' element which can be used on you both during antenatal classes and during labour are as follows:

- **Pelvic movement:** This involves constant response to pain signals and it consequently minimises the effect of anything which might otherwise impede the birthing process.

- **Making contact with the earth and becoming 'rooted':** See Figures 6.1 and 6.2. Striking these poses will allow you to make any tension flow out and for new energy to be drawn up from the earth, which will be concentrated in your belly area. This kind of exercise is strengthening and will give you a sense of purpose.

- **Combatant poses:** See Figures 6.2 and 6.4 (overleaf). These will allow strength from the 'earth' element to be used, as well as your will, which is part of the 'fire' element. The poses also facilitate your surrender to the 'water' element and your mastery of the 'air' element. They will activate your ability to make decisions and exercise your will and they will unify the passivity of the 'earth' element with the activity of the 'fire' element. To achieve these poses you will need to stand firmly on both legs, bending your knees (so that you can clearly feel your thighs); your pelvis will need to be tipped forward, your arms stretched up to eye level and held straight out, and your fists will need to be clenched; you will also need to look proud, decisive and focused. In this starting pose you will need to take a few deep breaths, then breathe in... and on the out-breath you will need to stretch your right leg outwards. Transferring your weight to this foot, while at the same time stretching your arms out to the right side too and shouting out 'Ha!' your left leg will be stretched out behind you, while your right knee is bent. You should breathe in as you return to the central position and then repeat the same turn towards your left side. This exercise will become even more powerful if you shout out 'I will!' while breathing out and turning to the right before saying 'Ha!'—and if you shout out 'I can!' whenever you turn to the left before saying 'Ha!'. If you do this exercise in a group, it should be done with everybody standing round in a circle and everyone moving in the same rhythm. This exercise will then serve not only to make you more aware of your own strength, but also to give you the feeling of collective strength.

- **Sitting poses:** The same effect can be achieved while sitting down, with your legs wide apart. You should slap your thighs hard while saying 'Aaaaaaah' and also repeatedly stretching out your legs, while also extending your fingers and making the sound 'Rrrrrrrraah!' While you are doing all this your eyes should be wide open and staring at the person sitting opposite you.

- **Eye exercises:** Doing eye exercises can also be a very effective way of stimulating the 'fire' element. At eye level, using the index finger you should trace figures of eight of varying sizes, while allowing your eye to follow the shapes that you trace, without moving your head while you do so.

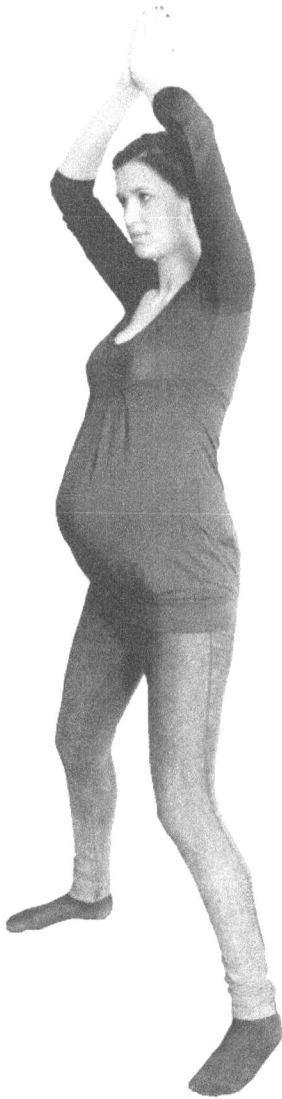

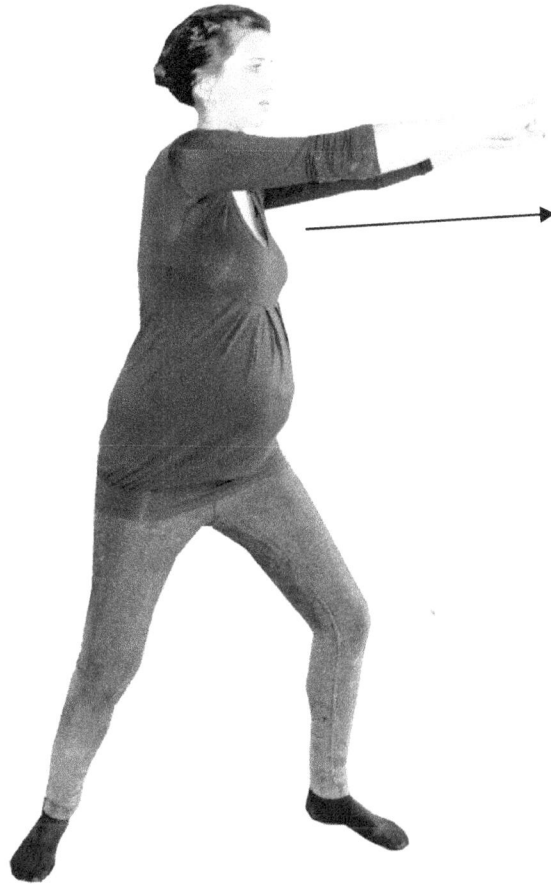

Figure 6.2

Figure 6.1

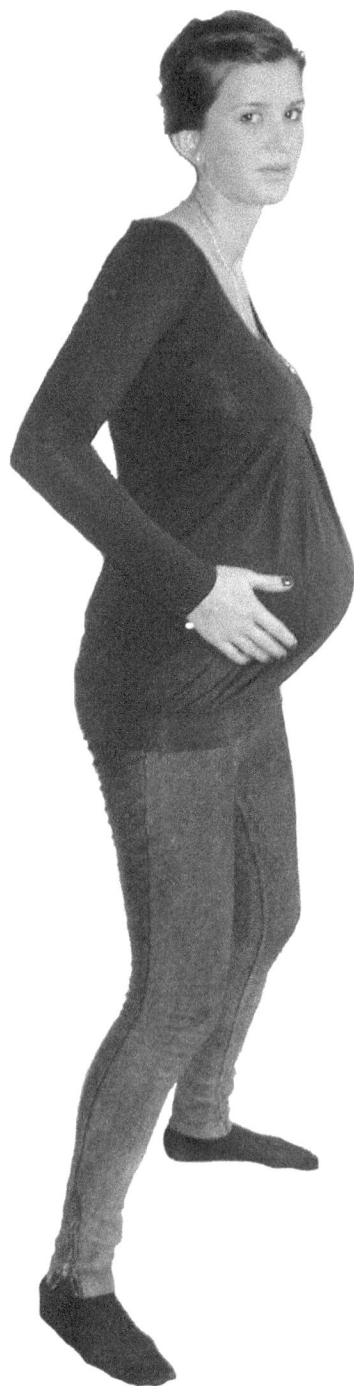

Figure 6.3

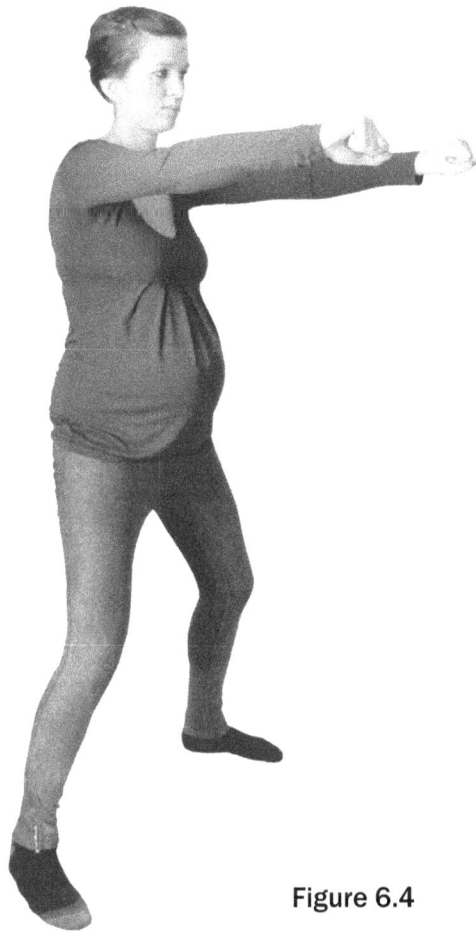

Figure 6.4

- **Fire dancing:** While listening to suitably fiery music, you should dance freely, stamping your feet, clapping your hands, bringing your thighs strongly into the dance, keeping your eyes wide open and maintaining eye contact. This is 'active relaxation'.
- **Active relaxation poses:** These are poses where you hold a 'rooted' position (as in Figure 6.3) with your muscles active (with a feeling of 'force in your body). This will allow your to release any tension and also recharge your energy. These poses will facilitate the natural flow of your labour by promoting in you an attitude of surrender (the 'water' element) in positions which support the work of your baby inside (i.e. by promoting 'active passivity').
- **Activating changing rhythms:** Between each phase of active or passive body work, to finish off you should always come to a position of rest in order to become 'rooted' again and tune back into your body.

WATER – THE LEVEL OF DEEP FEELINGS

The 'water' element symbolises surrender, receptive passivity, flow and sexual energy. This element accompanies any pain and makes it more effective in pushing the labour forward. It will enable an opening up of your ability to feel… an expansiveness; it will activate your parasympathetic nervous system and facilitie deep communication between you and the baby within you.

With the 'water' element your subconscious feelings and deep-down fears will gradually emerge and your intuitive sense will strengthen, as contractions become stronger and opening up occurs. The 'water' element will dissolve any resistance and allow the strong flow of contractions towards the birth itself by facilitating your surrender and capitulation. The less resistance there is in you, the less pain you will experience.

You will need to 'hold in' the 'water' element (i.e. contain it) if you are not to lose yourself in it completely. The spatial and human environment should serve the purpose of 'holding things in' (by acting as 'stops', giving you a sense of things being near and limited). This will allow the 'water' to flow into the sea.

In order to promote the 'water' element in your body it is necessary for your midwife or birth attendant to stimulate your breasts, pelvis and ankles. Ask him or her to use slow, flowing movements, pressing down, and alternate these with lighter, faster ones, always moving their hands downwards.

Visualisations

It is helpful for you to do visualisations, using metaphors which are very symbolic. The visualisations act in the following way:

- They will facilitate fast release. They will help you to become immersed in what's happening!
- They will activate the right-hand side of your brain and this will activate your neurovegetative, hormonal and emotional system.
- Visualisations will also strengthen your instinctual knowledge and trust.
- They will help you become united with nature and its elements and activate your life forces.
- They will help you to overcome blockages caused by fear and negative imprinting.

Sample exercises

- Visualise the water in your own body. See its depth, its colours, its ability to disappear and move. Also see the feelings in you that are linked to this water.

- Visualise your growing baby in its own, clear lake of water. Imagine what your baby looks like, how it is focused on the placenta which gives it everything it needs. Ask your baby questions. Share your thoughts with him or her. Make promises. Surround your baby with energy. Rock your baby using the rhythm of your breath…

Improving your sexual energy

During your pregnancy and while you are in labour, immersing yourself in the 'water' element will help you to feel trusting and to surrender yourself to the processes taking place. It will create the necessary intimacy which will allow you to open up emotionally and physically. It will dissolve any muscular tension and make it very easy for you to move around and adopt various poses. It will stimulate your sexual energy, which consists simultaneously of 'water' and 'fire' energy. Making all these things happen will facilitate the dynamics of your labour and the necessary opening up process. Sexual energy is the only energy which drives the birthing process. Exercises which bring your sexual energy to conscious awareness include the following:

- **Active body work** on the pelvic floor, coccyx and sacrum, to strengthen them and release tensions. Ask your partner to give you a massage and apply pressure or strokes to your body so as to 'activate' or stimulate the energy in your body and in that of your baby being born.
- **Light massage**—as in Figure 6.5. Ask your partner to hold his right hand on your sacrum/coccyx and his left hand on your neck or occiput. Breathing between his two hands will activate your woman's sexual energy and open up your pelvis.
- **Conscious passivity exercises** where you learn to consciously 'let things happen' while having contractions and in breaks between them.
- **Contrast exercises** where you learn the rhythm between being more active while having contractions and more passive in the pauses, when you listen deep within your self. Over time, you should experience greater contrast between the times of tension and times of release.

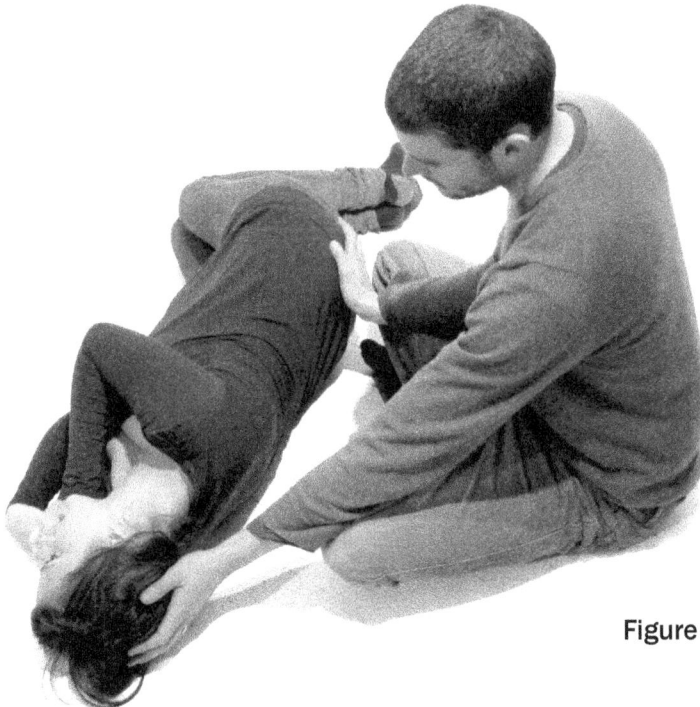

Figure 6.5

Sample exercises

- **Group contractions:** The group should stand round in a circle. (In classes involving couples, women and men should alternate around the circle.) Each person should become 'earthed' and should search out a good position to stand in. Each person should imagine that with each out-breath he or she is taking root. The breath can be seen as a colour. On the in-breath, the breath should flow over the roots back into the body. Each person should feel how, with each out-breath, the roots are spreading out and digging into the earth. Next, each person should reach out to the person standing on his or her right (his or her right hand should take the next person's left hand). Then each person should imagine that the in-breath is coming from the body of the person on his or her right, into his or her own body, and also that the out-breath is flowing into the body of the person standing on his or her left. During this visualisation each person should imagine a wave like movement around the circle, moving towards the left and round.

  Now, each person should imagine a 'contraction'... He or she should keep the left hand relaxed and tense up his or her right hand. Then he or she should breathe into the left hand and increase pressure on the right hand as the pain 'increases' and then slowly let it fade away. In the break between 'contractions' which follows, each person should focus on feeling the earth again, letting his or her breath flow down and out into the roots, letting it go and letting everything become soft. When the next 'contraction' comes each person should again imagine the breath coming from the person on the right and flowing over to the person on the left.

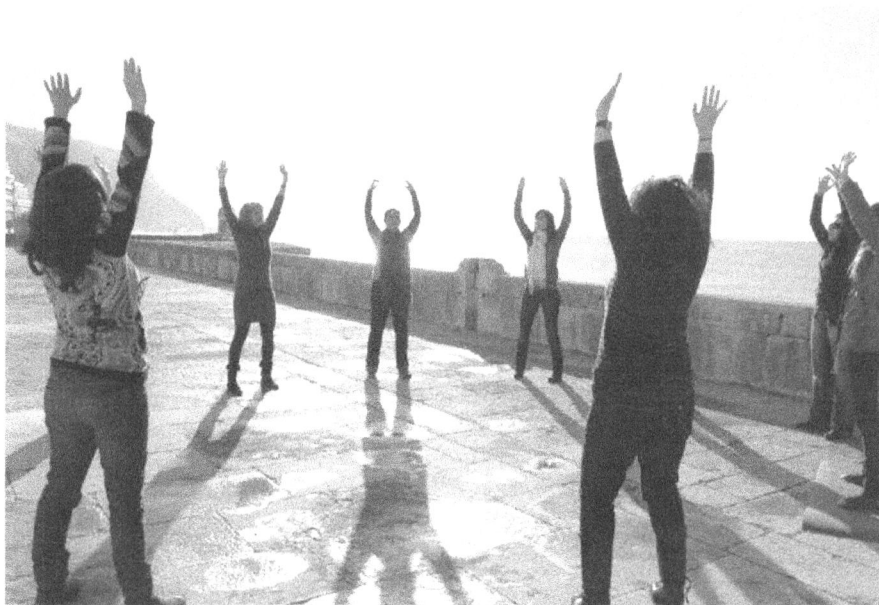

Here Verena leads some pregnant women through some other moves

These visualisations should be repeated using vocalisations (moaning) too. Pressing hard when tensing up your right hand, each contraction should last the same length of time as the breaks between 'contractions' (i.e. one minute). At the end of this exercise, you should let go of your neighbour's hands. You should then focus on how each hand feels. Does it feel bright, dark or colourful? Is it warm? Finally, you should all talk about how you found the exercise. You should then focus back on your pregnancy and your baby inside, who is not yet ready to be born.

- **Pelvic work:** This exercise should increase your perception and promote your awareness. Using pelvic circling (see Figure 6.6 overleaf), inspired by Feldenkrais (see www.feldenkrais.co.uk), the 'water' element in your pelvic area is gently brought into movement, without any 'water' slopping over the sides! While you are standing up or lying down on your side, your partner should use a tennis ball to make you aware of first one side, then the other side of your body. While you are standing or lying on your side, your partner should then work the tennis ball into your ischium, coccyx and symphysis. After this, while you are sitting up, the ball should be lain between the sides of your ischium; you should breathe out any pain or unpleasant sensations or deal with them by making vocalisations. Also help yourself to cope by seeking out useful images and ideas. Afterwards, you should talk about what you have felt and thought.
- **Water dancing:** In this exercise, you make gentle, sensual swaying movements, focusing on your chest and pelvis, so that you gradually open yourself up more and gradually feel more and more in touch with other people. This exercise will allow the 'water' element to start moving.
- **Pairwork:** Each person should massage his or her partner from the shoulder blades, over the shoulders, upper arms and then down to the hands.
- **Leg and foot massage:** With the goal in mind of making the 'water' element move (which is particularly useful if you are suffering from oedema), either your midwife or your partner should move your ankle and massage the arch of your foot. You should also make pumping movements with your feet, shake your legs, lift up your legs, rock your pelvis and stretch out your legs.
- **Working in threes:** Stand between two other participants and—as you breathe in—you should raise your arms high above your head. As you breathe out, you need to bend forward while also stretching your arms out to the front, holding your back straight. One of the other two people in your threesome then needs to pull your pelvis back, while the other person pulls your arms forward. You should then breathe deeply while your back is stretched in this way. The participant who is standing behind you should then massage you from the shoulders, down your back to your iliac crests (hip bones).
- **Singing:** This is very effective in stimulating the 'water' element. It will bring your feelings to the surface and harmonise them. Singing is also a good tool for expressing pain and is very useful for diminishing pain perceived, while also helping you to open up your cervix. It will calm down your unborn baby and strengthen your sense of connection with your baby.

EARTH – THE MATERIAL, PHYSICAL LEVEL

The earth is the level of sensitivity and cognition, of trust and courage, solidity, realisation and concentration.

The earth is about sensitivity and cognition, trust and courage, solidity, realisation and concentration

Your pelvic floor is the energy centre of the 'earth' element. The 'earth' element holds things firm, safeguards things from change... and is therefore also against any kind of opening up. Nonetheless, this is also the element of your growing baby. If the 'earth' element becomes too constricted your pain will increase and your labour will slow down. This element can reduce the amount of pain you experience when it works on the peripheral aspects of your pain— on physical aspects of your pain, for example when pressure is put on painful areas, when there is movement and bodily contact. This will allow your pain to be reduced.

In order to activate the 'earth' element in your body, your neck, the nape of your neck, your sacrum, pelvic floor, knees and feet need to be stimulated. Movements should be slow so that each stroke goes deep down into each part of your body.

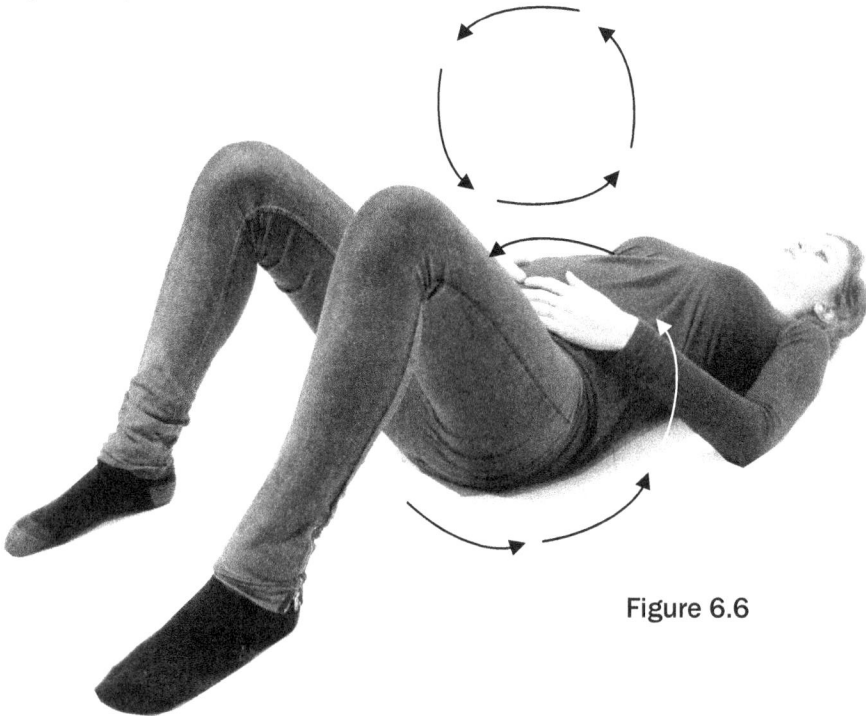

Figure 6.6

Sample exercises

- **Feeling the earth barefoot:** Finding a good position to stand in, you should first of all put your weight on one foot, then on the other. Then you should start walking, in slow motion, allowing each foot to make good contact with the 'earth' (the floor). You should tune into whether each foot is making good contact with the floor and slowly allow each foot to release this contact as you feel your balance shifting towards the other foot, taking strength from the earth as you place each foot down.

- **Taking root completely:** There are many ways of doing this... You can stand quietly, with your feet hip-width apart and knees slightly bent, with your back slightly tilting forwards. You can let the weight of your head sink down into your shoulders, then let the weight of your shoulders sink down into your pelvis, then let the weight sink further down to your knees, feet, right down until you feel as if you're sinking deep into the earth. Another way is for you to slowly put your weight onto one foot, keeping your knee bent and letting your foot 'take root' in the ground. Then you can tear yourself away from the ground and transfer your weight to the other foot, repeating this switchover several times; each time one of your feet makes contact with the floor your need to feel that you are growing deep roots. After doing this exercise you should put your weight evenly onto both feet and focus on how they both feel. Still another way of 'taking root' is to let your 'light' foot (i.e. the one which isn't carrying your weight) be brought round to one side of your body, at a 90 degree angle and then put this foot down on the ground in such a way that you feel you are growing deep roots. Then you need to bring this foot back round to the front, put it down, while transferring your weight to it, and then do the same with the other foot, the second time moving your other foot round to the other side of your body. Again, after this exercise, when in a balanced position, with weight evenly distributed on both feet, you should focus on how each foot feels. Doing this exercise should relieve any pain in your ileo-sacral joints.

There are many ways of helping you to 'take root'

- **Deep-breathing while lying down:** While lying down you need to feel that you are taking root at each point where your body is making contact with the ground. As you do this, you can focus on how there seems to be an exchange of energy between yourself and the earth... It needs to be as if sometimes you are giving yourself up to the ground and sometimes that you are drawing strength from it. You also need to focus on the feeling you have in your pelvic floor and breathe along with what you feel in that area.

You may be able to draw strength from the ground.
It will be helpful for you to breathe along with
what you feel in your pelvic area.

Another way of using the 'earth' element is through touch, with a midwife or birth partner using either pressure or massage.

Pressure and massage during pregnancy:

- While you are lying on your back, a tennis ball should be put on your sacrum. The ball should then be used to massage one side of your pelvis from the sacrum, to the iliac crest, moving from top to bottom. When any pain is experienced you should use your breath, as well as moaning and intoning. After a while, the ball should be taken away and you should focus on what you are feeling. After this, the other side of your pelvis can be gently massaged in the same way. During this massage, you can also visualise your own 'earth' element colour, i.e. you can focus on the colour(s) you experience on the right-hand side, and on the left. You should also consider how you are lying on the earth and how you feel about the person who is doing the massage... Where do you perceive the 'earth' element being in your masseur and what does it look like? What kind of space does it take up? (There can be many variations on this kind of question, of course.) Perhaps you can even describe or paint a picture of what you see afterwards.

- While sitting on the floor, you should draw your buttocks back, one by one. While doing this, you should be aware of your ischium, the trapeze-shape in your pelvis between the public bone and the coccyx (tailbone), and you should focus on how your ischium feels. Next you should breathe out... Then, on the in-breath which follows, you should feel your pelvic floor going towards the earth (or the floor). As you breathe out again, you should feel how your pelvic floor contracts into a central point, which is like a star. After this, you should sit on a tennis ball, so that it's in the centre of your ischium. Around this area, where you should feel pressure, you must relax fully. You should imagine images, make sounds and use your breath so as to cope with this. After doing this exercise, you should take the ball away, sit down again and focus on any sensations you are experiencing.

Pressure and massage for use both during pregnancy and labour:

- **Sacral pressure:** Ask your midwife or birth attendant to exert pressure on your sacrum (see Figure 6.7 overleaf).

- **Sacral stroking:** Ask your midwife or birth attendant to exert rhythmic pressure on your sacrum by stroking up and down (see Figure 6.7), following the rhythm of your contractions and the breaks between contractions—stopping stroking as each contraction passes and applying firm pressure during your contraction.

- **Whole body stroking:** Ask your midwife or birth attendant to stroke you all over your body (as in Figure 6.8).

- **Foot massage:** If your midwife or birth attendant massages your feet and particularly your little toes, he or she will stimulate the 'earth' element in you and strengthen it. (See Figure 6.9.) It is also possible for you to give yourself a self-massage using a tennis ball.

- **Polarity massage:** This involves massaging your sacrum and belly, while you lean against a wall. This has an analgesic effect. (See Figure 6.10.)

- **Pubic polarity massage:** This involves your midwife or birth partner putting one hand on your pubic bone and the other hand on the inside of your upper thigh while you breathe normally. (See Figure 6.11.)

- **Head and neck massage:** This is useful when you are exhausted from being in labour. Your midwife or birth attendant needs to put one hand on your head, and the other on your feet.

- **Pelvic floor massage:** In this case, your midwife or birth attendant firmly massages along the edges of your ischium.

- **Partner contact:** Loving touch from your partner, might well help you to cope and open up.

- **Pelvic floor work:** Your midwife or partner can actively work on your pelvic floor as a basis for body work.

- **Feet:** Your midwife or birth partner can actively work with your feet, help you to feel roots and move your sacrum.

- **Head and neck:** If you move your head round in circles you can release and relax your neck (as in Figure 6.12).

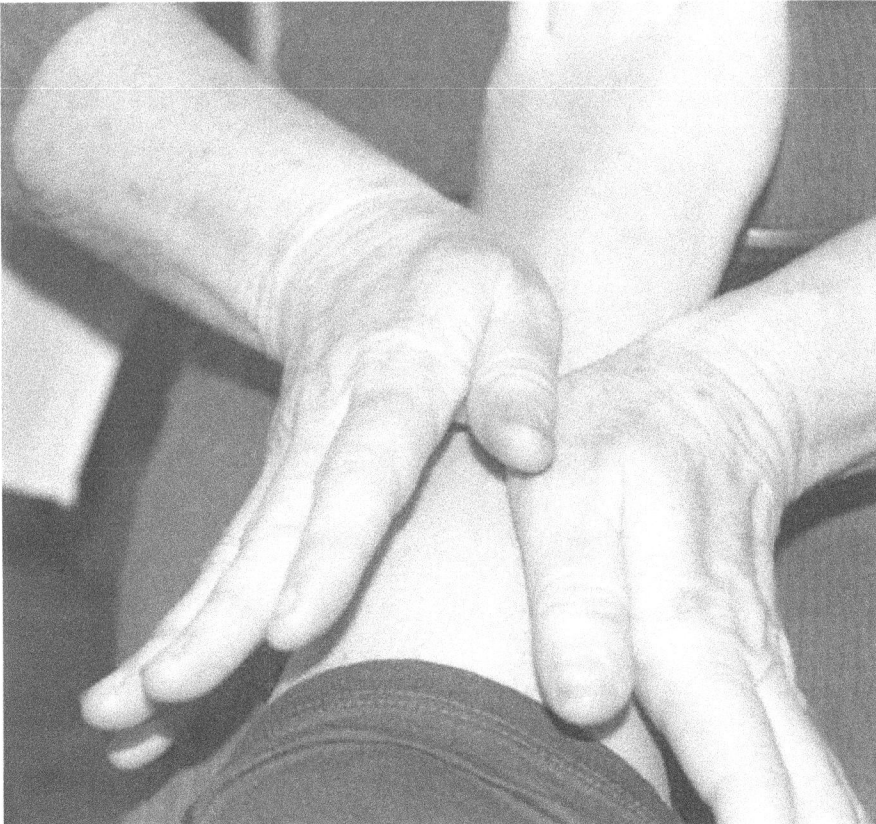

Leg and foot massage can be very helpful

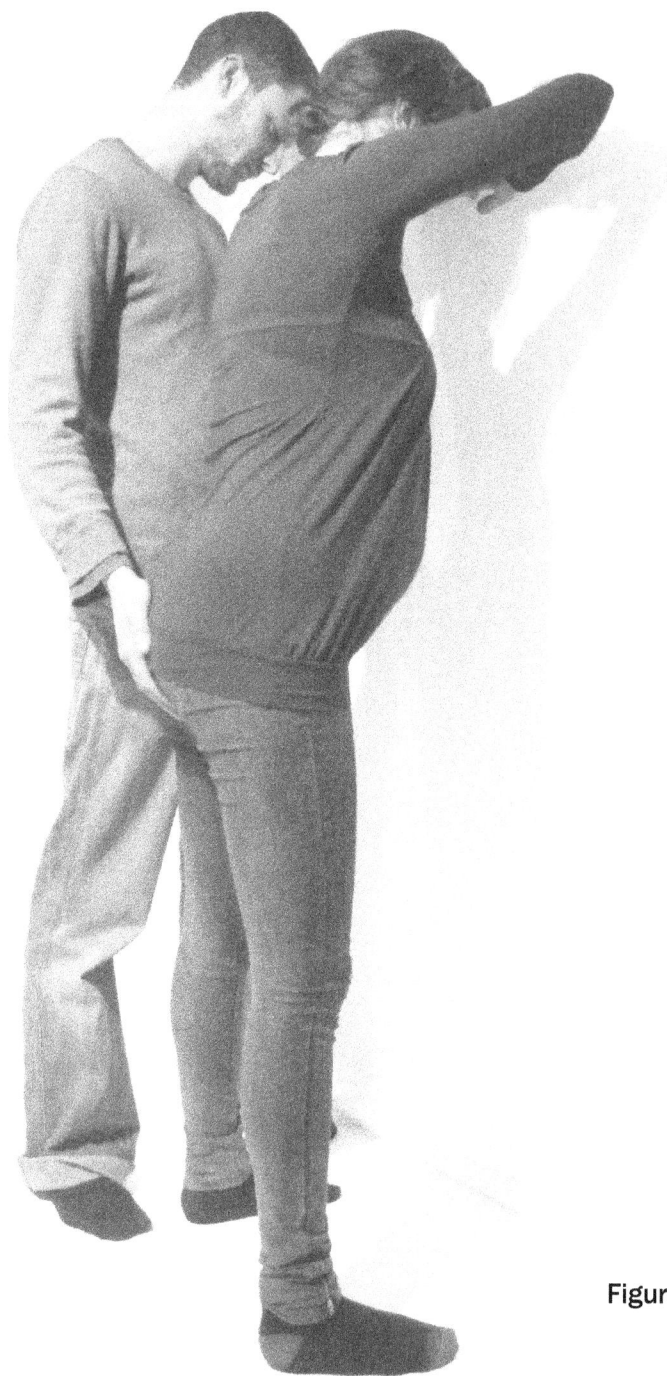

Figure 6.7

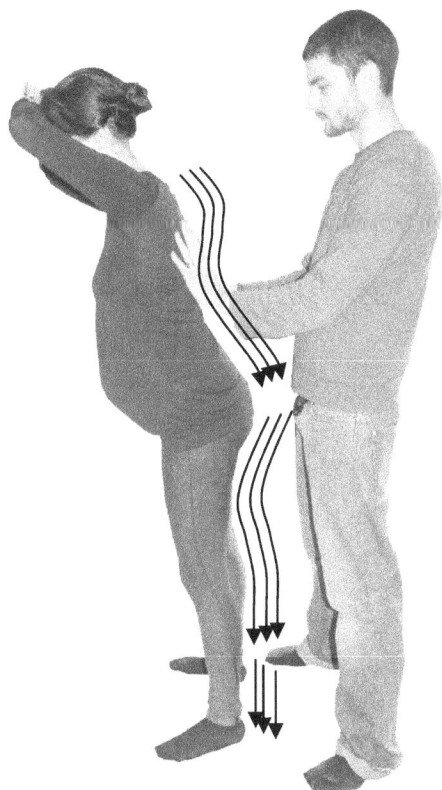

Figure 6.8

Figure 6.9

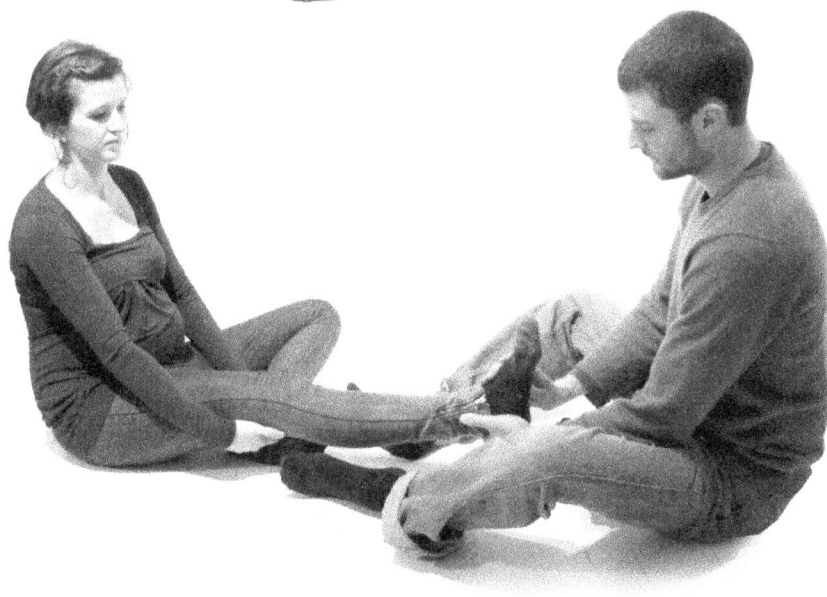

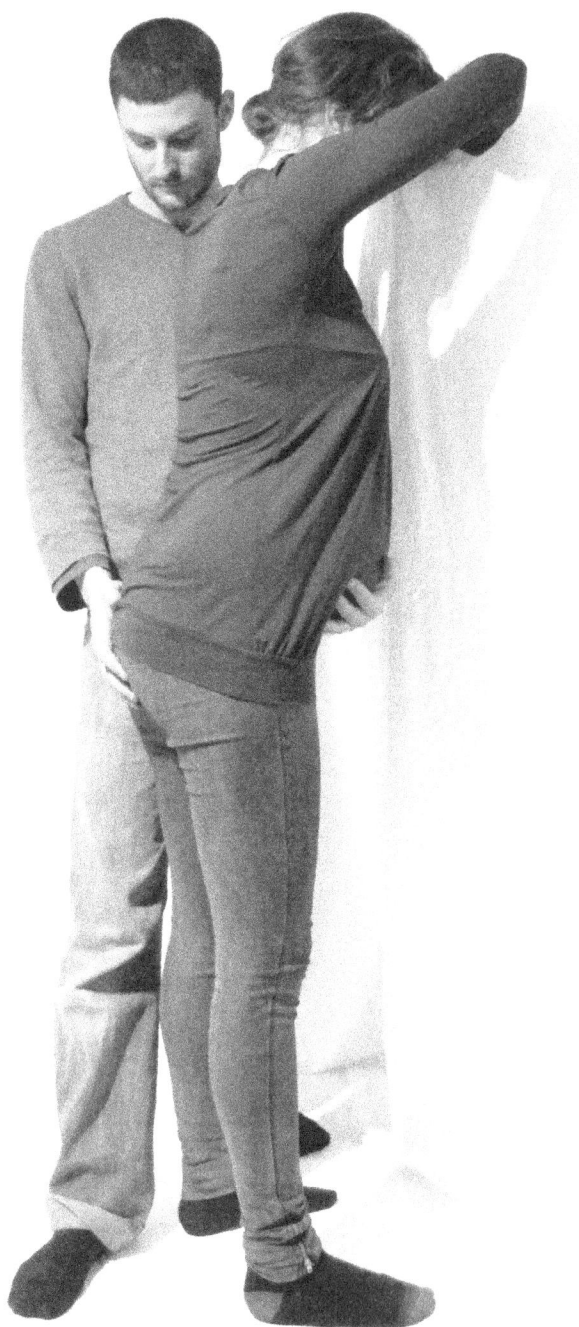

Figure 6.10

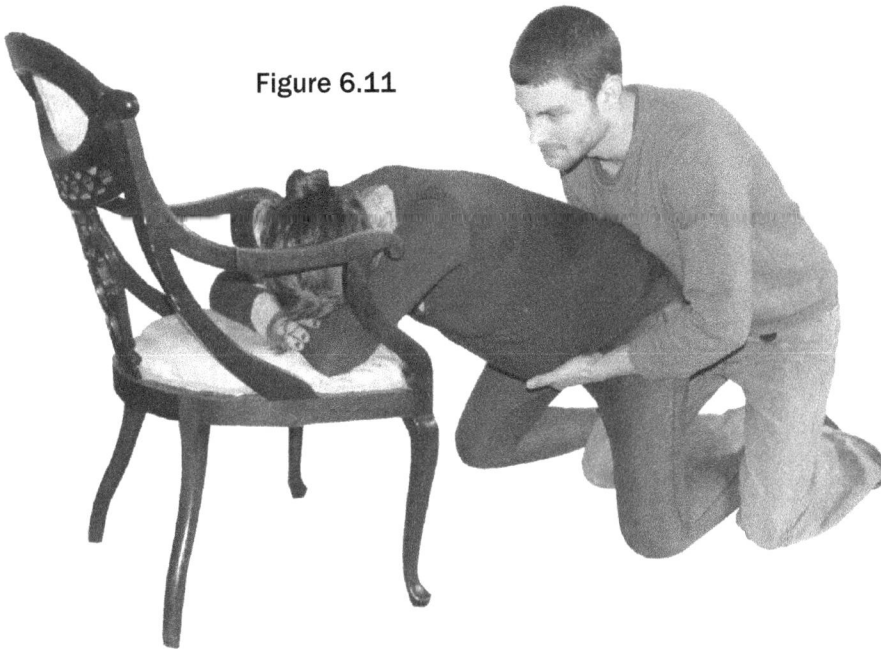

Figure 6.11

AIR – THE SUBTLE, MENTAL AND SENSORY LEVEL

Air is the level of adaptation and flexibility, which comes along with movement. The most important tool for stimulating this element during labour is the breath. This can also be one of the most effective means of pain relief.

During labour, the 'air' element can have an inhibitive effect in that it increases the perception of pain, as long as it remains in the mental dimension, in your cortex. However, when its presence in your mind is stimulated through the senses (e.g. using aromatherapy, light movement or music) it can actually promote the other elements and your adaptation to the various phases of labour. Breathing during birth is the most important expression of the air element and the most effective tool for dealing with pain.

Breathing is a physiological function which can be both voluntary and involuntary and as such it can bridge the gap between our conscious and unconscious mind (i.e. it can transmute 'air' to 'water'). In this way your breath can give you access to your unconscious (i.e. it will activate the 'water' element). Specific breathing techniques will influence the chemistry in your brain and can therefore change your level of consciousness.

A deep and slow in-breath, which brings air deep into your abdomen, followed by a slow out-breath will be effective in giving you a sense of well-being during your pregnancy. During labour this kind of deep, controlled breathing can release tension and activate your parasympathetic nervous system.

In order to activate the 'air' element in your body, it is necessary to stimulate your arms and shoulders, your kidney region (by making circles with your hips and bending over), as well as the calves of your legs. Your movements should be gentle, fast, superficial and should go in all directions—and then they will have a suitably 'cleansing' effect. At the same time it is important for you to feel 'well-grounded' on the earth, so that you can keep your balance and not drift away.

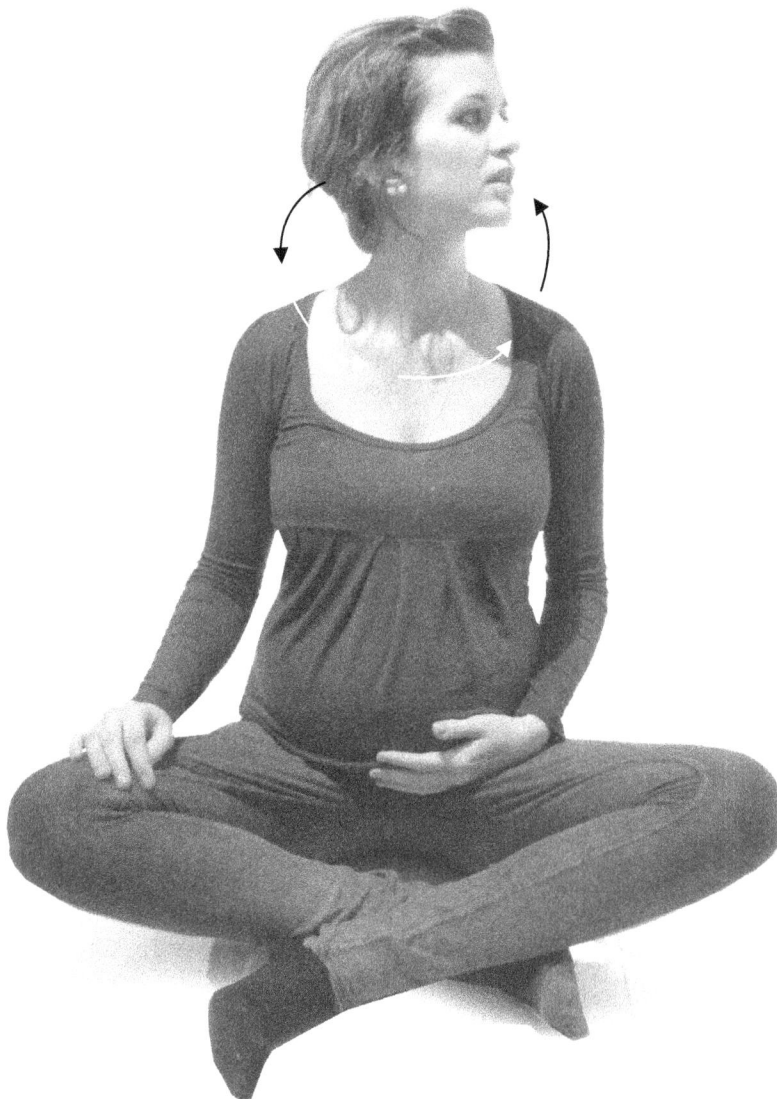

Figure 6.12

Sample exercises

- **Slow out-breaths:** These breaths are active and open you up, in order to release any tension. They will help you to become connected with the earth and they will activate your parasympathetic nervous system and stimulate the production of endorphins, while also reducing your exertion (which results in the production of lactic acid). Slow out-breaths will also help to bring the 'air' element in the direction of the earth and they will give you a sense of peace and well-being.

- **Passive in-breaths:** Deep breathing will have the effect of facilitating your movements, provided you breathe in harmony with your movements.

- **Long out-breaths focusing on a specific part of your body which you voluntarily contract:** If, while breathing out, you focus on releasing tension from a particular part of your body (for example your contracted fists or your her feet), this will help you to relax.

  Long out-breaths for reducing pain: Breathing out can be a way of making tension (which results in pain) tolerable. This exercise needs to be done with a partner (as in Figure 6.12). You start by lying on your back, either with your hands comfortably positioned behind your head or with your arms stretched out on either side of you (to the right and the left). Draw your right leg up (so that your foot is as close as possible to your bottom), while your other leg remains outstretched. Then ask your partner to help you to very gently put pressure on your bent leg (at your knee), so as to bring this to touch the floor on the other side of your body respecting your limits (i.e. without forcing your limits). While your partner does this keep your shoulders firmly on the floor (perhaps with your partner helping to hold them down) and twist your spine round. Note that although you will initially be briefly on your back, during the exercise you will actually be lying on your side.

- **Long out-breaths while focusing on painful or tensed up parts of your body:** Make long out-breaths while you are focusing on an area which is painful or tense (perhaps because of a contraction, or because of pain in the lower segment of your uterus). On your long out-breath you should also use your voice (intoning or groaning), to help you cope with the pain.

- **Air dancing:** Light, cheerful music can be used. Dance around using silk scarves, changing partners often if you are dancing in a group. If you are dancing with a partner sometimes you should be leading and sometimes you should fit in to what other people are doing.

- **Work on your spinal column:** Any work on your spine will improve flexibility (i.e. your ability to move around) and your ability to adapt to what is going on within your body. (See Figure 6.14 overleaf to see an example of this kind of work.)

During a drug-free labour free, spontaneous breathing, movement and vocalisation will help you to refocus on the intensity and dynamics of the labouring and birthing process. Your free and spontaneous expression will be disturbed if anybody gives you any instructions or commands. If your labour is difficult, breathing, movement and vocalisation will be important therapeutic methods of pain relief.

Figure 6.13

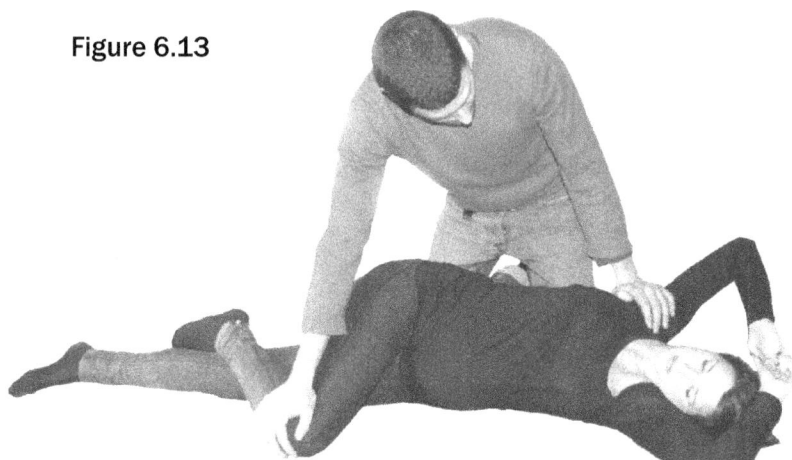

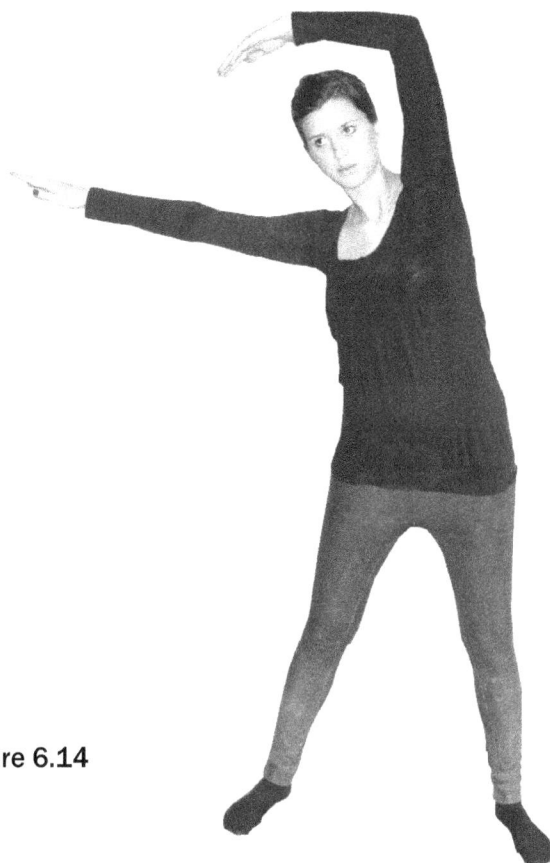

Figure 6.14

VOCALISATION

Using your voice...

- will help you to lengthen and lighten up your out-breaths
- will produce profound vibrations which will help to reduce your pain
- will open up your pelvis and your pelvic floor and release muscular tension
- will stimulate your body to produce endorphins
- will activate the 'water' element (since it will help you to express your feelings and your subconscious thoughts)

SINGING

Using your voice in a musical way...

- will activate the 'water' element, bring your feelings to the surface and harmonise your expression of pain
- will have a strong pain-reducing effect and help your cervix to dilate
- will calm and strengthen the baby inside you
- will allow you to express joy and lightness of being when you use your voice alongside the 'air' element

DANCING

Moving round rhythmically...

- will allow you to feel a sense of lightness and well-being
- will activate the elements and thereby all levels of your body and all feelings which are connected with your 'pain' in any way
- will help you to slip into your own rhythm and find your own way of expressing yourself physically
- will play an important role when you are experimenting with different possibilities and learning about yourself
- will rock your baby

POLARITY THERAPY

Various relaxation techniques can be used to harmonise the elements and also reduce any chronic stress and thereby prevent this from leading to pathology. A universally applicable approach is Polarity Therapy, which was originally developed by Dr Randolph Stone. Born in Austria in 1890, he later emigrated to the USA and devoted himself to studying natural healing, chiropractic and osteopathy. He brought together the teachings of Ayurvedic medicine, yoga, traditional Chinese medicine and the Egyptian and Greek philosophies of medicine and finally concluded that a 'life energy' lies at the heart of all states of being and that this 'life energy' is constantly flowing between polarities. (This energy is called *chi* or *prana* in other systems.) He was talking about a kind of subtle electro-magnetic energy. We can think of this force as a kind of circular field of energy, which circulates around our body and surrounds it. Just like electricity, it is thought that this energy flows from a positively charged pole to a negatively charged one.

If your midwife or a birth partner engage with the currents of your life energy they can help your energy to flow more and they can bring it into a state of balance. When this energy is flowing freely you will feel good, balanced, calm and healthy. There is no 'bad' or 'good' energy... only well or poorly directed strength. Polarity Therapy will bring this life force back into its natural channels by dissolving 'energy knots' (caused by physical or emotional stress). As soon as this blocked up energy is released, it will meet your specific needs at any particular moment, according to the laws of physical self-regulation.

In order to be able to correctly understand the principles of this therapy and use it effectively your midwife or birth partner will need to go on a course to study Polarity Therapy. However, there is also a simple form of Polarity Therapy which can be used during pregnancy and labour, so as to have a positive effect on your life energy. It will stimulate your parasympathetic nervous system and thereby make you relaxat and it will also promote inner communication between you and your baby. It will also help you to perceive your own deep needs. If your midwife or birth partner can make use of this therapy, they will be able to prevent stress-related pathology or treat it when it occurs. This is possible because Polarity Therapy will allow help them to be devoted and attentive and to spoil and support you, while they are busy doing beautiful things. It will also help you to remain in communion with your baby, amongst other things. These are all things which tend to become increasingly forgotten in everyday life, since it is filled with duties, or they are relegated only to the realm of the sick. So make sure somebody who is helping you learns about Polarity Therapy!

Another very helpful aspect is work on energy channels in your pelvis and pelvic floor, which is possible with Polarity Therapy. Even during labour, using this therapy, in a short time it is often possible to easily correct malpresentations of the fetal head or to positively influence dynamic or mechanical forms of dystocia (i.e. failure to progress). In addition, it is possible to achieve a remarkable reduction in pain perception by dissolving tensions which cause pain, promoting a deep state of relaxation during the breaks between contractions. In this way, your pain will be reduced to a physiological minimum, so you will find it easier to tolerate it. As a result, your experience of birth will remain 'intact'.

Beyond this, Polarity Therapy is even believed to help your baby, help it overcome the stress of labour and birth and help it to more easily adapt to being in its new world. In my experience, it also makes it possible to positively influence various problems which might arise after the birth such as an inadequate milk supply, depression and an accumulation of lochia (postnatal discharge), which is due to subinvolution of the uterus.

The simplicity of using movement and positioning of the hands allows a deep effect to take place. Your midwife or birth attendant will only be able to learn this method of treatment through experience, after a basic grounding in Polarity Therapy generally.

A sample Polarity Therapy session

You lie comfortably on your left side. Your Polarity Therapist e.g. your midwife) will need to sit or kneel comfortably behind you (having removed jewellery, watches and mobile phones). She will then place her left hand on you (while you're still pregnant, or when you're already in labour), in the hollow between your collarbone and your shoulders. Next she will need to put her right hand on your sacrum, making sure that her fingers are lying on your ileosacral joints and that her little finger is on your coccyx. Both of her hands should lie flat, but not be laid heavily on you. Next, she will take her time to make contact and to tune into the spontaneous movements underneath her hands, letting her breath flow freely. Then she will imagine that she is allowing her breath to stream between her two hands, so that a 'breath circle' is created (flowing up through her arm, across her shoulders, down through her other arm, through one hand positioned on your body over to the other, in a circle, or, if it is easier, only between her two hands). She will allow sufficient time for it to be possible to imagine this developing. When the breath is finally circulating on its own (without any effort on her part), she will support the flow of energy by finding a rhythmic way of moving her hands, one by one, alternating between light rocking and calmly tuning in. (Each time she feels the energy pulsing through her fingers, she will gently rock that hand again.) Alternating rocking with tuning in, she will eventually feel heat or pulsating or other signs of energy flow. To finish off the process, she will hold her hands still, just imagining the breath circulating. At the end of the Polarity Therapy session, she will take her hands very, very slowly off your body.

Polarity Therapy is a deeply relaxing treatment and it can also be combined with another procedure which is good for reducing pain during a contraction

This one procedure constitutes a deeply relaxing treatment, but it can also be combined with a second procedure, which is particularly good for reducing pain during a contraction. The second procedure involves leaving the therapist's right hand in its original place on your sacrum, with her left hand seeking out a good place on your lower belly above your pubic bone on the lower segment of your uterus (as in Figure 6.9). The rest of the procedure is as before... Again the therapist will make good contact with her hands, she will tune into any sensations coming from your body. The breath will begin to circle round and when necessary her right hand will rock lightly for a while, alternating with pauses in which the therapist will tune into what is happening afterwards, under her hands. To finish off this treatment, the palms of both her hands will be lifted from your sacrum and lower belly and lain upon the soles of your feet (slowly applying a steady, increasingly firm pressure) and they will be left there to have an effect. As before, the treatment will conclude when the therapist's hands are gently and slowly lifted from your feet.

8: Develop your own ways of coping

Consider other ways of learning about pain

These are many ways of learning about pain and how you can deal with it. Consider what suits you and the methods you want to use during your labour. The important principles for preparing for labour involve the following steps:

- Share knowledge about the meaning of pain so that you feel motivated to face it.
- Find out about tools for coping with pain in different birthing settings so that you feel you will be able to cope with the pain of labour.
- Remember that symbols are a very effective and fast way of reaching deep inside you and helping you to feel and understand your feelings. Nevertheless, every kind of body work can be adapted to your needs in labour so as to help you face normal labour pain.
- Offer your partner support and help him understand how he will be able to support you during your labour and birth.
- Get used to the idea of reacting to pain in physiological ways, i.e. through spontaneous, instinctual movement and by expressing your feelings using your voice (i.e. singing or making sounds).
- Make long out-breaths so as to release tension and relax more effectively.
- Make your body flexible, particularly in the pelvic region.
- Strengthen and train your pelvic floor area (e.g. by doing Kegel exercises).
- Channel your body's energy through your body (down your spine and legs, using your breath)—i.e. use the male force.
- Learn how to relax and let go completely in the pauses between contractions—i.e. use the female force.
- Learn the importance of the rhythm between tension and relaxation during contractions and the breaks between each one.
- Get someone to give you massage and other treatments during your pregnancy because this will help you discover what might be most helpful for you during your labour.
- Realise that the efforts you make during your pregnancy and labour will lead you towards a gratifying goal.

When you understand what is going on, when you can orient yourself to the process of labour and birth, when you feel you have some tools to cope with labour, when you know your own resources and when you understand the deep meaning of the process for you and your baby, then you will be able to face the experience of birth and you will trust the healthy processes which are taking place, which are all leading you towards the point when you will at last meet your baby.

When you understand the process of labour and birth, you will be able to face it

CHAPTER 7:

Opening up to your baby and coping with pain

The process of childbirth

In *Birth Without Violence* (Wildwood House, 1975—republished by Inner Traditions, 2002) Frederick Leboyer writes about the process by which a labouring woman lets go and gives herself up to the process of birth. He compares the opening up process of birth to what happens when a person falls in love. In that situation a person is happy to just open up and let things happen. He says that if you just allow yourself to open up, an enormous power is unleashed so as to bring your baby into the world. It is a kind of surrender, he says, which will allow you to let go of your baby and release him or her into the world, so that this tiny person can take up a new life.

In my view, the cause of labour pain is negative evaluation of the experience of birth. In other words, it is your aversion to the idea of letting go of your baby, which in itself represents a division of part of your self. In order to allow this division to take place, it is necessary for you to completely open up to your baby, physically and emotionally, so as to be able to accept it and let it grow into being. The process of opening up can take place in various ways: gently through a gradual opening which even begins during pregnancy, forcefully through intensive pain during labour, through ongoing suffering postnatally due to the baby's unexpected needs, or even through later pain and suffering.

It's possible your unborn baby remains as yet unknown to you as a separate person. Perhaps you experience your baby simply as an object or as a body, which grows inside you up to a certain size, which you perceive as being either too big or too small. If this is the case, birth will certainly be a difficult process, because you will feel you need to open yourself up to allow your body to produce a strange, unknown 'thing' which will significantly influence your life in the future too. If you feel this way, you will naturally have a sense of aversion and resistance.

But what if your unborn baby is in a dialogue with you and what if there is a continuous exchange between both of you? If this is the case, you will receive whatever messages your baby sends you and get to know his or her personality. You will begin to understand what it is like to experience a reciprocal relationship, and will start to perceive your baby's special characteristics. You will learn that both you and your baby need to work together in the process of birth, and also that your baby is contributing to your common goal with his or her own strength and personality and helping you too, just as you are helping your baby. If you understand this, you should be more able to open yourself up to your baby.

Opening up to your baby means listening and opening up to yourself... giving up all resistance.

Opening yourself up to your baby means listening and opening up to yourself, to your deep inner self and to the life inside you. Opening up to the life inside you means giving up all resistance: resistance to life with its particular rhythms, resistance to pain and joy, to the unexpected, to change and also to necessity. Opening up means meeting the demands of life head on. It means that you will need to give yourself up to the flow of your biological and spiritual power, trusting yourself and your body and having a positive vision, just as you would in a sexual relationship. If you open up and give yourself up to the processes going on within you, you will then be able to meet the challenge of birth alongside your baby—harmoniously and cooperatively.

Separation and disengagement become far easier when you realise that your baby is a separate person, when you know who you will meet and hold in your arms, after completing the work of birth. In short, you will be able to open yourself up to your baby when your resistance is minimal because your pain will then also be reduced to a minimum.

If you have minimal resistance, your pain will be minimised

The process of emotional opening up needs to take place in advance of any physical opening so as to make that physical opening up possible. Furthermore, the process of opening needs to continue over a long period of time: while your abdomen is swelling during pregnancy, while your cervix is dilating, during the first stage of your labour, as well as while you are breastfeeding after the birth. In order for the appropriate kind of opening up to take place safely, your need to be treated with respect at all times and people around you will need to help you establish safe boundaries. Your relationship with your partner should make you feel safe and respected, so you should feel able to communicate within this familiar and protective environment, as well as with your midwife or to other caregivers.

In the final analysis, opening up to your baby even during your pregnancy is the most important and effective of your resources when it comes to reducing the pain of your labour and transforming any sensations—whether neutral or painful—into ecstasy.

Like any other all-embracing concept, this concept of opening up is not just about the moment of overcoming pain during the actual birth; it goes far beyond that. It applies to all areas of your personality and should dramatically change all inner and outer interconnected systems.

You need to open up on all levels

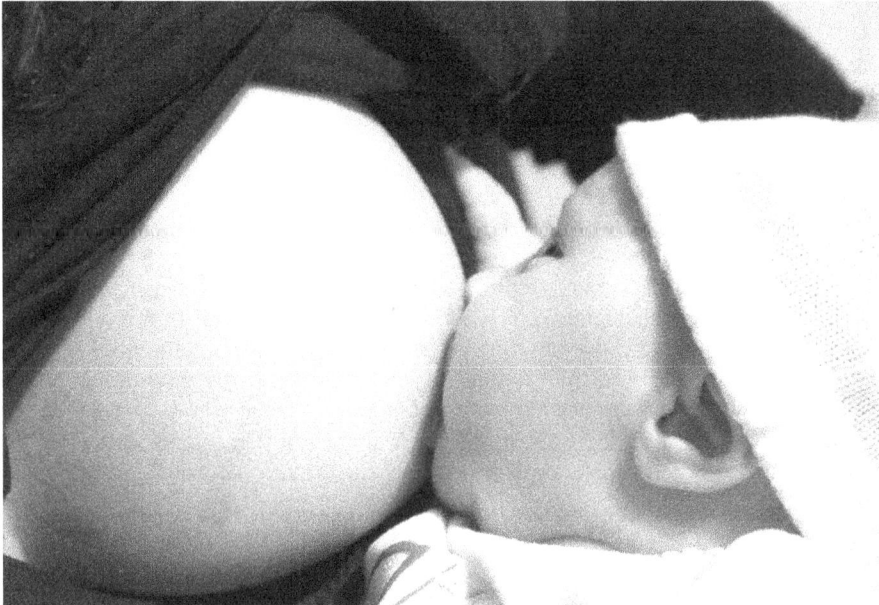

Photos © Sandro Pintus

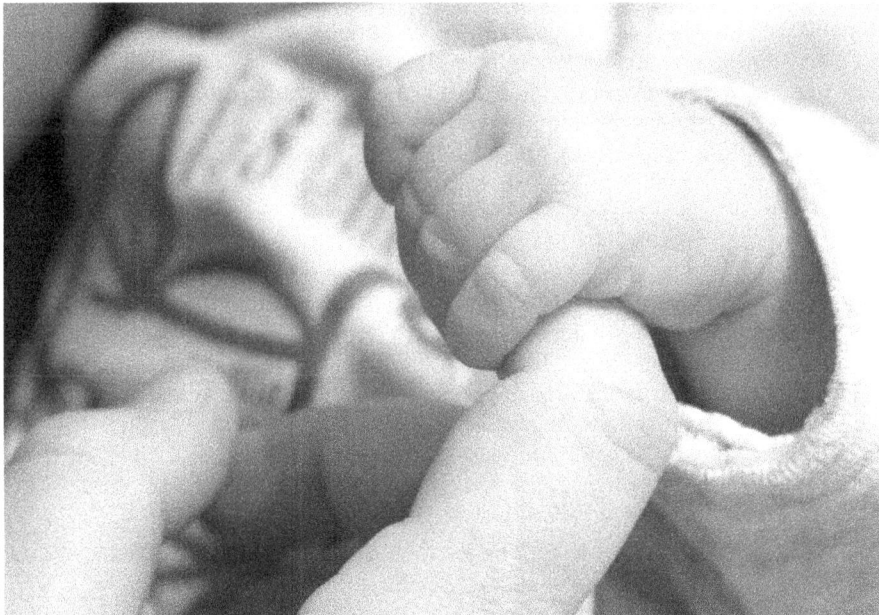

Opening up to your child, is absolutely vital if you want to facilitate the processes of birth and early motherhood, whether the baby is still inside you or in the world outside your womb, breastfeeding or snuggling up to you

Your own decisions about pain relief

After finding out about pain in labour and postnatally, and after obtaining information about all methods of pain relief available to you, you should be able to make your decisions about your own labour. Your midwife should help you do this by providing professional, non-authoritarian, but empathetic, accepting, all-embracing care, which will involve—whenever necessary—guiding you, perhaps with your partner, through labour, birth and through parenthood generally.

When considering how you are going to cope with labour and open up successfully to the processes going on within you, remember that any kind of opening up is likely to make you feel vulnerable. This means it's important that you find support in the form of a midwife (or other caregiver), who will listen to you sensitively, help you communicate and support you in preparing for labour. This person should:

• help you to accept your vulnerability and become increasingly self-aware.
• help you confront the unknown, make deep contact with yourself and use archaic forms of communication, such as intuition and ancient wisdom.
• help you to open up, go deep inside yourself and develop an archetypical understanding of your baby.

In order to find an appropriate person, look for a midwife who appears to know herself well. If she does, she is likely to be capable of differentiating between herself and the women for whom she is providing care. When a midwife does not understand her own problems with womanhood and motherhood and her own fears and limitations, and when she is not aware of her talents and special capabilities, she will tend to project her own wishes and preconceived ideas onto you. As a result, she will expect you to behave in a certain way and that will influence your decisions. Above all, when a midwife does not understand her own problems she is not usually in a position to tolerate or support the expression of pain. Often the request for some kind of pain relief will be triggered by a care provider, and not from you yourself... This is because the midwife—or other care provider, or your birth partner—cannot stand hearing you express your pain and cannot bear its strength. In this way, it is possible for you to be brought to the point where you request pain relief or accept it when it's offered by the people who are attending you in labour, simply because the other people present are reminded of their own pain and their inability to bear it! When you're in labour it's as if you can see, written all over your caregivers' faces: "That must really be terrible—quite horrific!"

If you want really want to experience labour and birth as you've decided you want to experience it, you will need to find a midwife (or consultant) who is in tune with and supportive of your choices. You need to understand the meaning and function of any pain you will experience. Unless you recognise its potential to transform you, you will quickly begin to seek out ever more powerful forms of pain relief... but remember that this may mean you are only effectively *deferring* the opening up process not escaping it. Whatever choices you make, remember the potential of the pain to help you develop.

Keep away from people or situations where you find impatience, intolerance, fear and the need to 'do something', when it's not really necessary or helpful for either you or your baby. Don't allow any caregivers to insist on any kind of treatment or intervention (e.g. to accelerate your labour and birth), just so that they can escape their own fear. You have the right to refuse and protect the integrity of both your own and your baby's body.

If you make your decisions about pain relief yourself, you will be able to travel through the profound and existential process of childbirth more easily and become engrossed in its emotional aspects... Cherish this process, as you will not have the opportunity to go through it many times in your life.

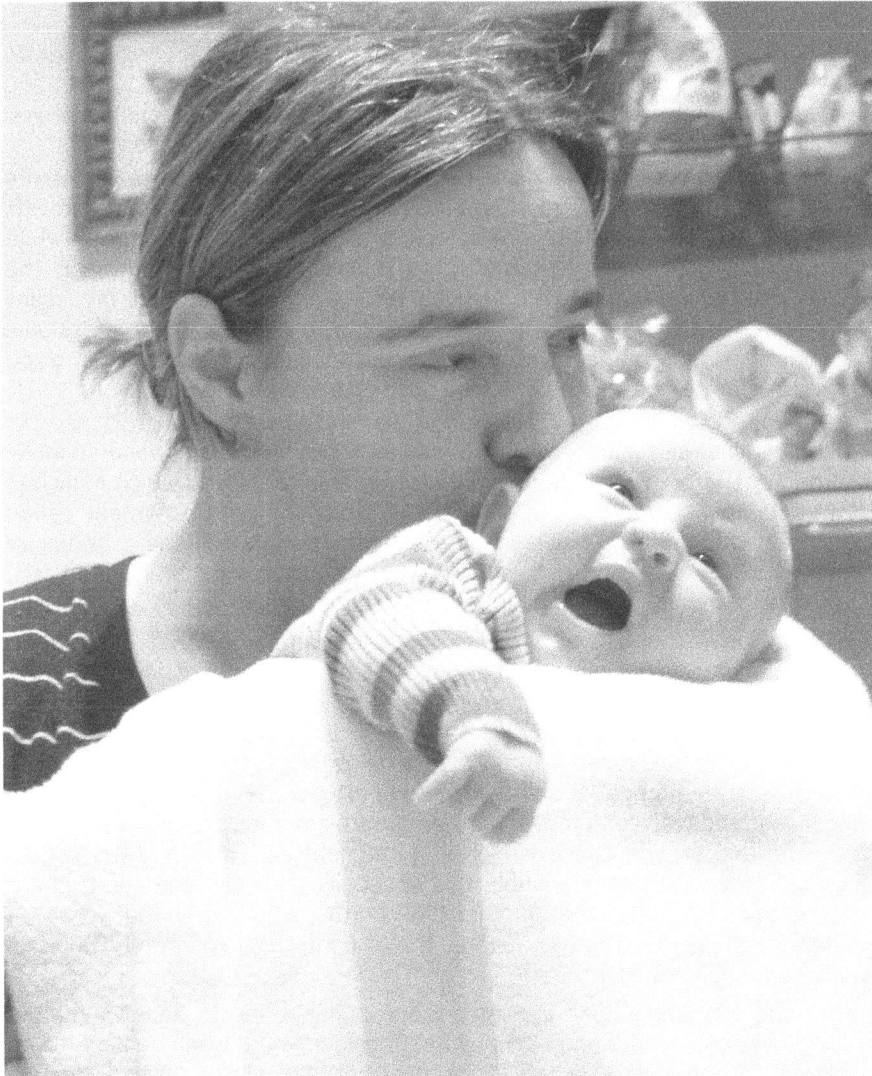

Photo © Sandro Pintus

Remembering the conditions necessary for natural pain relief

Taking into account the wider reasons we have discussed for valuing pain in our lives and recognising that pain in childbirth may have a specific important function in our lives, you may use your freedom of choice to opt for a birth with no—or minimal—drug-based pain relief. If you experience an entirely physiological birth, i.e. a birth with no drugs or interventions, you may well experience childbirth as empowering. You may also find that it is a key to your own personal development, because this may well be facilitated as a result of your experience of giving birth.

In order for this to happen, you will be wise to remember the conditions necessary for natural pain relief to be possible...

- Find a stable and trustworthy care package. This means finding a midwife who offers her clients support in all phases of pregnancy, labour, birth and also postnatally, within the context of a professional relationship. If you cannot find this on the NHS, consider hiring an independent midwife.
- In order to reduce your fear and pain and increase your trust, your midwife will need to make you feel safe. She will also need to be ready to provide you with any appropriate physiological or psychological support, while facilitating your empowerment. Within a care team, your midwife is the professional who can most effectively facilitate the eventful life processes which take place around the birth of a baby, and she is the professional who is best placed to support women's health in general—so make sure you find a midwife who you feel will fulfil this important function.
- If you are looking for a midwife within the NHS, note that you may need to contact your local Supervisor of Midwives so as to find someone suitable. The Supervisor of Midwives should also be able to tell you which midwives in your local area work in teams and which operate a system called 'caseload midwifery', which means that one midwife will see a particular client all the way through pregnancy, birth and the postnatal period. You may also want to go to www.birthchoiceuk.com to check out your options.

After you have found a supportive midwife, remember that even when individual midwives are motivated to engage with the model of care described here, which involves the minimisation of physiological pain, they sometimes quickly confront the limits of what they can do in their particular working environment. For this reason, it may also be wise for you to secure the services of a doula, or to arrange for another trusted birth partner to be with you during your labour and birth—either your partner or a trusted friend or relative. A doula is trained and experienced in supporting pregnant and labouring women, so should be fairly comfortable within this situation. The most important thing—whether you have a doula or another birth partner with you—is that you have continuous support during your labour. This is particularly important if you feel at all fearful about the birth.

Beyond this, remember the importance of labouring in an environment which feels safe, secure and very private. Consider where it will be best to you to give birth—whether at a large maternity hospital, at a midwifery-led unit (within a large hospital), at a birth centre, or even at home.

Your choices, your birth, your new start in life...

With the right preparation, after making conscious decisions based on your perceived needs, with appropriate support during labour, labouring in an appropriate place, you should easily find the courage and motivation to have the kind of birth you want for yourself. Opening up to your baby will become a major part of your life... a rewarding and fulfilling experience. Most importantly, you should be ready to meet your new baby with confidence and joy.

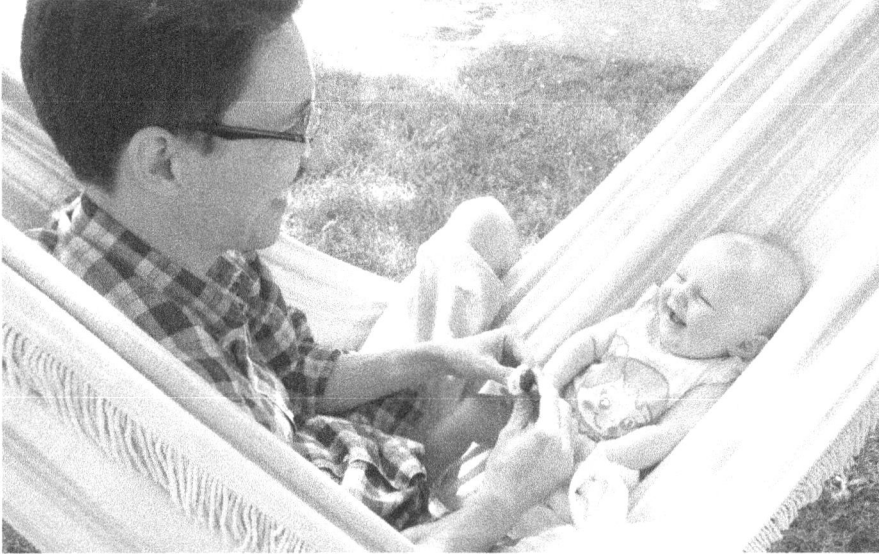

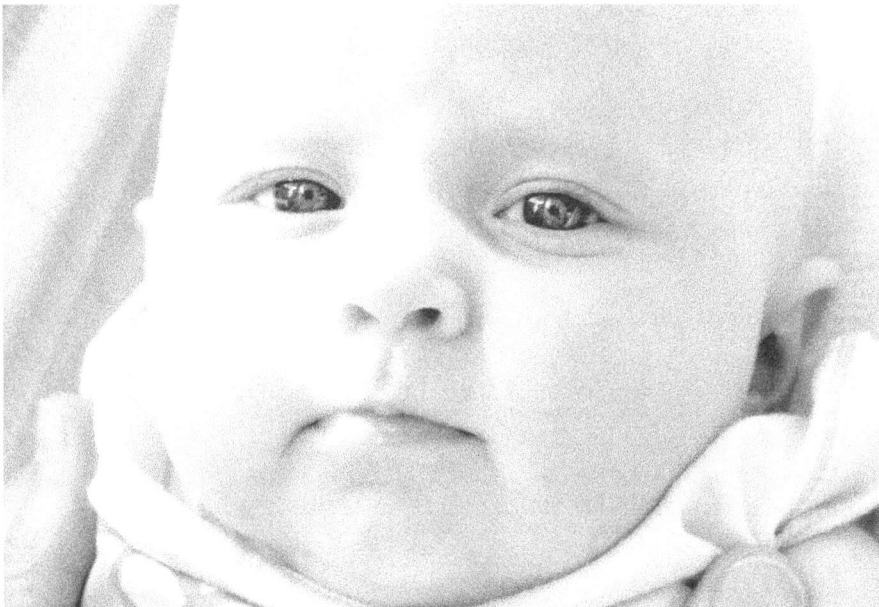

Photos © Sandro Pintus

Bibliography

Agnetti B, *et al*, 1997. *Ipnosi e Autoipnosi in Gravidanza.* Bonomi, Italy.

Agnetti B, 1992. *L'Ipnosi Medica nel Parto.* Grasso, Italy.

Anderson T, 2002. The misleading myth of choice: the continuing oppression of women in childbirth. MIDIRS, Vol 12, No 3, Sept, pp 405-407.

Antony MA, Stein MB, 2008. *Oxford Handbook of Anxiety and Related Disorders.* Oxford, USA.

Arms, S, 1994. *Immaculate Deception II: Birth and Beyond.* Celestial Arts, USA.

Arms, S, 1975. *The Immaculate Deception.* Houghton Mifflin Book Company, USA. (Note this book is now out of print but the sequel above, *Immaculate Deception II: Birth and Beyond,* is still available.)

Balaskas, J, 1994. *New Active Birth. New Active Birth.* Harvard Common Press, USA.

Baumann G, *et al,* 2002. Le donne scelgono il parto cesareo? *Donna e Donna, il giornale delle ostetriche*, No 38, Sept.

Bedwell C, Dowswell T, Neilson JP, Lavender T, 2010. The use of transcutaneous electrical nerve stimulation (TENS) for pain relief in labour: a review of the evidence. *Midwifery,* Feb 17. [Epub ahead of print]

Beech B, 2000. Over-medicated and under-informed, what are the consequences for birthing women? *AIMS Journal*, Vol 11, No 4, Winter.

Bing E, 1967. *Die Lamaze Methode.* Marion von Schroeder Verlag, Germany. (The updated edition is as follows: Lothian, J and DeVries, C, 2005. *The Official Lamaze Guide: Giving Birth with Confidence.* Meadowbrook Press, USA.)

Bonica, JJ, 1977. *Anestesia e Analgesia in Ostetricia.* Il Pensiero Scientifico Editore, Italy.

Bottaccioli, F, 1997. *Psiconeuroimmunologia.* Red ed, Italy.

Brackbill Y, Kane J, Manniello RL, Abramson D, 1974. Obstetric premedication and infant outcome. *Am J Obstet Gynecol.* Feb 1; 118(3): 377-84

Bratteby LE, 1981-9. Effects on the infant of obstetric regional analgesia. *Journal of Perinat Med.* Suppl 1:54-6.

Buckley S, 2005. *Gentle birth, gentle mothering.* One Moon Press, Australia.

Buckley S, 2005. The hidden risks of epidurals. *Mothering*, No.133, Nov-Dec.

Buxton CL, 1962. *A study of psychophysical methods for relief of childbirth pain*. Saunders, USA.

CeVeas (Centro per la valutazione dell'efficacia dell'assistenza sanitaria), 2004. *La Sorveglianza del Benessere Fetale in Travaglio di Parto: Linee Guida Basate sulle Prove di Efficacia*. CeVeas, Italy. (Website: www.saperidoc.it)

Chertok L, Langen D, 1968. *Psychosomatik der Geburtshilfe*. Hippokrates Verlag, Germany.

Clement S, 2000. Psychosocial outcomes with different modes of delivery in Royal College of Midwives. NCT (National Childbirth Trust). In 'The rising caesarean rate: causes and effects for public health.' Conference Report No 7, Nov, London, UK.

Collis RE, Davies DW, Aveling W, 1995. Randomised comparison of combined spinal-epidural and standard epidural analgesia in labour. *Lancet*, Jun 3;345 (8962):1413-6.

Davis, E, 2000. Women's sexual passages. Hunter House Publishers, USA.

Davis-Floyd R, 1992. *Birth as an American Rite of Passage*. University of California Press, USA.

Dick-Read G, 1993. *Childbirth Without Fear*. Harper & Row, USA. (This book was re-published by Pinter & Martin in 2007.)

Dodwell M, 2002. Should women have the right to a clinically unnecessary caesarean section? *MIDIRS*, Vol 12, No 2, June, pp 274-277.

Donati, *et al*, 2001. Valutazione dell'attività di sostegno e informazione delle partorienti: Indagine nazionale. Istituto superiore si Sanità, Rome, Italy. (Website: www.saperidoc.it)

Donati S, Andreozzi S, Grandolfo ME, 2001. *Valutazione dell'attività di sostegno e informazione alle partorienti: indagine nazionale*. Rapporti ISTISAN 01/5. Istituto Superiore di Sanità, Rome, Italy, pp 20-21.

Ehrenreich B, English D, 1973. *Witches, Midwives and Nurses.* Feminist Press, USA.

Enkin M, Keirse M, Neilson J, Crowther L, Hodnett E, Hofmeyr J, 2000. *A Guide to Effective Care in Pregnancy and Childbirth.* Oxford University Press, UK. (Updates are available via www.cochrane.org.)

Erickson MH, 1967. *Advanced Techniques of Hypnosis and Therapy.* Grune & Stratton, USA.

Filippini MN, 2007. *Donne Sulla Scena Pubblica.* Edizione a Stamp, Italy.

Filippini N, 1995. *La Nascita Straordinaria Tra Madre e Figlio—La Rivoluzione del Taglio Cesareo.* Franco Angeli Storia, Italy.

Friedman D, 1974. Parturiphobia. *American Journal of Obstetrics and Gynecology,* 118:1, 130-135.

Gadsby JG, Flowerdew MW, 2000. Transcutaneous electrical nerve stimulation and acupuncture-like transcutaneous electrical nerve stimulation for chronic low back pain. *Cochrane Database Syst Rev,* 2000(2):CD000210, Update in *Cochrane Database Syst Rev,* 2006;(1):CD0010.

Gaskin IM, 1978. *Spiritual Midwifery.* Book Publishing Company, USA. (Note, this is now available in its fourth edition, which was published in 2002.)

Gaskin, IM, 2008. *Ina May's Guide to Childbirth.* Vermilion, UK.

Gibbins J, Thomson AM, 2001. Women's expectations and experiences of childbirth. *Midwifery,* Vol 17, No 4, Dec, pp 302-313.

Giddens A, 1991. *Modernity and Self-Identity. Self and Society in the Late Modern Age.* Polity Press, UK.

Giddens A, 1992. *The Transformation of Intimacy: Sexuality, Love and Eroticism in Modern Societies.* Polity Press, UK.

Gordon R, 1978. *Your Healing Hands—The Polarity Experience.* Unity Press, USA.

Goria L, Cellana A, Basso M, 2001. Parto cesareo parto indolore? *Donna e Donna, il giornale delle ostetriche,* No 32, Mar.

Haire D, 1985. *The Cultural Warping of Childbirth.* International Childbirth Education Association, USA. (This is the reprint of a report carried out in 1972.)

Hannaford C, 2002. *Awakening the Child Heart*. Jamilla Nur Publishing, Hawaii.

Hannaford C, 2008. Manual from the workshop: The physiological basis of educational kinesiology. Unpublished

Hewitt J, 1986. *The Complete Relaxation Book: A Manual of Eastern and Western Techniques.* Rider, UK.

Hildingsson I, *et al,* 2002. Few women wish to be delivered by cesarean section. *BJOG, International Journal of Obstetrics and Gynecology*, Vol. 109, No 6, June, pp 618-623.

Hodnett ED, 2001. Continuity of Caregivers for Care During Pregnancy and Childbirth. Cochrane Review, Cochrane Library, Issue 3, UK.

Howell CJ, Kidd C, Roberts W, Upton P, Lucking L, Jones PW, Johanson RB, 2001. A randomised controlled trial of epidural compared with non-epidural analgesia in labour. *BJOG*, Jan;108(1):27-33.

Illich I, 2005. *Disabling Professions.* Marion Boyars, USA.

Istituto Superiore di Sanita, Rome, 2000. *Politiche per la Nascita nel 2000: Analisi Epidemiologica e Organizzazione dell'Assistenze.*

Jacobsen B, Nyberg K, *et al*, 1988. Obstetric pain medication and eventual adult amphetamine addiction in offspring. *ACTA Obstet Gynecol Scand*; 67;677-682.

Jacobsen B, Nyberg K, *et al*, 1990. Opiate addiction in adult offspring through possible imprinting after obstetric treatment. *BMJ*; 301:1067-70.

Jolly J, Walker J, Bhabra K, 1999. Subsequent obstetric performance related to primary mode of delivery. *British Medical Journal of Obstetrics and Gynaecology,* 106, pp 227.

Jordan B, 1992. *Birth in Four Cultures: A cross-cultural investigation of childbirth in Yucatan, Holland, Sweden and the United States.* 4th edition, Waveland Press, USA.

Kelly M, Johnson E, Lee V, Massey L, Purser D, Ring K, Sanderson S, Styles J, Wood D, 2010. Delayed versus immediate pushing in second stage of labor. *MCN Am J Matern Child Nurs*, Mar-Apr;35(2):81-8.

Khan KJ, Stride PC, Cooper GM, 1993. Does a bloody tap prevent postdural puncture headache? *Anaesthesia*. Jul;48(7):628-9.

Kitzinger S, 1985. *Women's Experience of Sex: The facts and feelings of female sexuality at every stage of life.* Penguin Books, UK.

Kitzinger S, 2008. *The New Pregnancy and Childbirth.* Dorling Kindersley, UK.

Kotaska AJ, Klein MC, Liston RM, 2006. Epidural analgesia associated with low-dose oxytocin augmentation increases cesarean births: a critical look at the external validity of randomized trials. *Am J Obstet Gynecol.* Mar;194(3):809-14.

Leboyer F, 1979. *Inner Beauty, Inner Light.* Collins, UK.

Leighton, B.L., and S.H. Halpern. 2002. The effects of epidural anesthesia on labor, maternal, and neonatal outcomes: A systematic review. *American Journal of Obstetrics and Gynecology* 186: S69-77.

Lesser MS, Keane VR, 1956. *Nurse-Patient relationship in a hospital maternity service.* Mosby, USA. (Out of print.)

Levine PA, 1997. *Trauma-Heilung.* Synthesis Verlag, Germany.

Lieberman, E., and C. O'Donoghue. 2002. Unintended effects of epidural anesthesia during labor: A systematic review. *American Journal of Obstetrics and Gynecology* 186: S31-68.

Martensson L, Stener-Victoorin E, Walling G, 2008. Acupuncture versus subcutaneus injections of sterile water treatment for labour pain. *Acta Obstet Gynecol Scand*; 87(2): 171-7.

Mayberry LJ, Clemmens D, De A, 2002. Epidural analgesia side effects, co-interventions, and care of women during childbirth: A systematic review. *American Journal of Obstetrics and Gynecology,* 186: S81-93.

Mead M, 2001. *Male and Female.* Harper Perennial, USA. (Originally published by Morrow in 1949).

Melzack R, Wall PD, 1989. *The Challenge of Pain.* Penguin USA.

Melzack R, 1973. *Puzzle of Pain.* Penguin, USA.

Mercer J S, Erickson-Owens D A, Graves B,Mumford Haley M, 2007. Effect of Maternal Analgesia on Newborn Transition in *Evidence-Based Practices for the Fetal to Newborn Transition. J Midwifery Womens Health.* 2007;52(3):262-272, Elsevier Science, USA.

MIDIRS, 1997. Informed choice for professionals: epidural pain relief during labour. MIDIRS and NHS Centre for Reviews and Dissemination.

Moore CD, *et al*, 1977. Transcutaneous electrical nerve stimulation does not relieve labor pain. Updated systematic review. *Obstetrics and Gynec.* Vol 9, No 3, Sept, pp 195-205. Also referred to in the abstract and commentary by Terry Coats, midwife. MIDIRS, 1998, p 64.

Newton N, 1987. The fetus ejection reflex revisited. *Birth*, 14: 106-108.

Noble V, 1991. Shakti Woman: Feeling Our Fire, Healing Our World—The New Female Shamanism. Harper, USA.

Nyberg K, 1993. Studies of perinatal events as potential risk factors for adult drug abuse. Thesis, Dept of Clinical and Alcohol Addiction Research, Karolinska Institute, Stockholm, Sweden.

Oakley A, 1986. *From Here to Maternity: Becoming a Mother.* Penguin, USA.

Odent M, 1993. *Primal Health Research Newsletter,* Vol 1, No 1, Summer.

Odent M, 2007. *Birth and Breastfeeding.* Clairview Books, UK.

Odent M, 2007. *Primal Health: Understanding the critical period between conception and the first birthday.* Clairview Books, UK.

Odent M, 2004. *The Caesarean.* Free Association Books, UK.

Odent M, 1987. The fetus ejection reflex. *Birth.* 14:104-5.

Odent M, 1999. *The Scientification of Love.* Free Association Books, UK.

Owen MD, D'Angelo R, Gerancher JC, Thompson JM, Foss ML, Babb JD, Eisenach JC, 1998. 0.125% ropivacaine is similar to 0.125% bupivacaine for labor analgesia using patient-controlled epidural infusion. *Anesth Analg.* March; 86(3):527-31.

Paciornik M, 1982. Come Partorire accoccolate, PISA ed, Italy. (Originally published as: Redecouvert Chez les Indiens: Apprenez l'accouchement accroupi; la meilleure position naturelle pour vous et votre enfant. Editions Pierre-Marcel FAVRE, France, 1982.)

Parvati Baker J, 2001. *Prenatal Yoga and Natural Childbirth*. North Atlantic Books, USA.

Parvati-Baker J, 1987. *Conscious Conception: Elemental Journey Through the Labaryth of Sexuality.* North Atlantic Books, USA.

Pescetto G, 1974. *Manuale Clinico di Ostetricia e Ginecologia.* Societa Editrice Universo, Italy. Also see the 2009 edition of the same book.

Piscicelli U, 1972. *Training Autogeno Respiratorio.* Piccin ed, Italy.

Rapisardi G, 2001. La nascita da taglio cesareo: e diverso per il neonato? *Donna & Donna*, No 32, pp 26-27. Centro Studi Il Marsupio, Italy.

Reich W, 1942. *The Discovering of the Orgone: 1. The Function of the Orgasm.* Orgone Institute Press, USA.

Relier JP, 2001. *L'Aimer Avant Qu'il Naisse.* Editions Robert Laffont, France.

Rich A, 1976. *Of Woman Born: Motherhood as experience and institution.* Norton, USA. Republished by Norton in 1996.

Robertson A, 1994. *Empowering Women.* ACE Graphics, Camperdown, Australia.

Robertson A, 1997. *The Midwife Companion: The art of support during birth.* ACE Graphics, Camperdown, Australia.

Rockenschaub A, 2001. Gebären ohne Aberglauben. Facultas Univ. Verlag, Germany.

Rockenschaub A, 1998. *Gebaren Ohne Aberglauben: Eine Fibel der Hebammenkunst.* Aleanor Verlag, Germany.

Sandal J, 2002. The national sentinel cesarean section audit report: what have we learnt and what do we still need to find out? *MIDIRS*, Vol 14, No 1, Mar, pp 78 - 83.

Schmid V, 2007. *Salute e nascita, la salutogenesi in gravidanza*, Apogeo ed, Italy.

Schmid V, 2010. *Apprendere la maternità*, Apogeo ed, Italy.

Schmid V, 2000. I sistemi fisiologici di adattamento e le risorse endogene. *Donna e Donna*, No 29, June 2000.

Schmid V, 2002. Il parto sicuro, *Donna e Donna,* No 38, Sept.

Stone R, 1986. *Polarity Therapy: The Collected Works I.* Book Publishing Company, USA.

Stone R, 1988. *Polarity Therapy: The Collected Works II.* Book Publishing Company, USA.

Taylor SE, 2002. *The Tending Instinct: How Nurturing is Essential to Who We Are and How We Live.* Times Books, USA.

van der Spank JT, Cambier DC, De Paepe HM, Danneels LA, Witvrouw EE, Beerens L, 2000. Pain relief in labour by transcutaneous electrical nerve stimulation (TENS). *Arch. Gynecol. Obstet.* 264:131–136.

van Gennep A, 1909. *Les Rites de Passage.* (Also available in a 1960 edition, published by the University of Chicago Press, USA.)

Various authors, 1989. *Prima Le Donne e I Bambini.* Guerini e Associati, Italy.

Various authors, 1999. La scelta informata, No 25, *Donna e Donna*, CSM ed, Italy.

Wagner M, 2001. Fish can't see water: the need to humanize birth. *Int. Federation of Gynecology and Obstetrics*, 2001 (MIDIRS JUN 2002)

Wagner M, 2000. *Bad Habits: A poor basis for medical policy.* AIMS Journal. Vol 11, No 4, Winter.

Walsh D. 2002. Fear of labour and birth. *British Journal of Midwifery,* 10, 2002, p 78.

Weil S, 1950. *Attente de Dieu.* Editions du Vieux Colombier, France.

World Health Organization (WHO), 1996. Care in Normal Birth: a practical guide. Report of a technical working group.

Index

Also available from Fresh Heart:

For you...

- *Birth: Countdown to Optimal...* information and personal accounts to help you prepare for the best possible birth (by Sylvie Donna)
- *Surprising, Inspiring Birth*: accounts of birth to inform, amuse and reassure (Sylvie Donna, ed.)
- *Birthing Normally After a Caesarean or Two*—a look at the evidence, as well as individual women's experiences (by Hélène Vadeboncoeur)
- *Birth Your Way*—information if you want to give birth at home or in a birth centre (by Sheila Kitzinger)

For your caregivers...

- *Optimal Birth: What, Why & How*—a reflective, narrative approach based on research evidence (by Sylvie Donna)
- *Birth Pain: Explaining Sensations, Exploring Possibilities*—the companion book, for midwives, to this book (by Verena Schmid)
- *Welcoming Baby*—a consideration of neonatal care (by Debby Gould)
- *Promoting Normal Birth: Research, Reflections & Guidelines* (by various authors—an international collaboration)

See the website for info and prices. All books can be bought online, or from any other online store (e.g. Amazon), or ordered through your local bookshop.

Other books by Verena Schmid...

in Italian:

- Bringing a child into the world: life paths through birth (*Venire al mondo e dare alla luce, percorsi di vita attraverso la nascita*). 2005, Milan, Italy: Apogeo Editions.
- Health and childbirth: salutogenesis in pregnancy (*Salute e nascita, la salutogenesi in gravidanza*). 2007, Milan, Italy: Apogeo Editions.
- Learning about maternity: the new challenge today to balance nature and culture (*Apprendere la maternita: le nuove sfide di oggi tra natura e cultura*). 2010, Milan, Italy: Apogeo Editions.
- This book in Italian: *Il dolore del parto: una nuova interpretazione della fisiologia e della funzione del dolore, per la donna moderna* (Childbirth pain: a new interpretation of physiology and the function of pain for modern woman). 2000, Florence, Italy. Centro Studi Il Marsupio.

in other languages:

The book *Il dolore del parto* (for midwives) is available in German and Spanish.

About the author

Originally from Switzerland, Verena Schmid moved to Florence in Italy when she was 18 years old. She initially trained and worked as a nurse for 10 years, before retraining as a midwife after starting her own family. Her first son was born in hospital when Verena was 26 and she also fostered a 6-year-old girl at that time.

After qualifying as a midwife, along with four of her colleagues, Verena decided to start attending home births. This was the first home birth practice in Italy. Two years later, Verena and some other midwives founded an organisation to continue promoting home birth in Italy. A year later, Verena had her own first home birth when she had her second daughter.

Over the next few years, while continuing to attend home births, Verena worked in a state-run family health centre and also taught antenatal classes. Then, in 1985, Verena started working independently and founded the organisation *Il Marsupio* (*The Baby Carrier*). Within a few months, she set up a centre in Florence (also called *Il Marsupio*) for women and couples who wanted to birth and raise their children naturally. The centre offered pregnancy care, antenatal classes and support during labour (including home birth care and/or support for women who wanted to have an active, conscious birth in a hospital or birthing centre), as well as postnatal care. The same year Verena took the opportunity to travel to Amsterdam so as to spend two months working with Dutch midwives.

At the age of 40, with many years of nursing and midwifery experience behind her, Verena started offering courses in the 'art of midwifery' at the *Il Marsupio* centre. These courses, which were designed for qualified midwives, provided a year of study and included various topics relevant to midwives, including birth preparation and female psychology. The centre regularly offered a range of short professional development courses.

From 1991-3 Verena again started studying herself, concentrating this time on Polarity Therapy and counselling. At the end of her course she founded the first specialist magazine for midwives in Italy, which was—and still is!—called *Donna e Donna* (*Woman To Woman*).

In 1996 Verena decided to set up a school to teach the art of midwifery— the Scuola Elementale di Arte Ostetrica. Founded with seven other experienced homebirth midwives from different parts of Italy, this was the first midwifery school in Europe run *by* midwives *for* midwives. From then on, Verena set up various national and international seminars and conferences, some of which have been taught by other tutors from other parts of Europe, North America or Mexico. At that point , Verena also started writing books...

Right: *Verena Schmid with her pregnant daughter, Anna Lou, and daughter-in-law, Carlotta, who is holding her three-month-old baby*

Until the publication of this book, Verena's work was not readily available in English. In her writing Verena has focused mainly on natural birth, both at home and in hospital settings, and labour pain. This book is hopefully the first of many available to English-speakers in Britain and America, and worldwide.

More recently, as well as continuing to write and teach, Verena has developed hospital-based courses for midwives, for continuing professional development. (These courses have been made available free-of-charge for individual midwives.) She has also campaigned for improvements in the law for both midwives and pregnant women in Italy, and continued her own studies—this time learning about 'focusing'. (This psychotherapeutic term describes a way of paying attention unjudgementally to specific sensations in the body, i.e. to something which is directly experienced, but not yet articulated in words.) In the year 2000, Verena received the International Astrid Limburg Award for her commitment to promoting independent midwifery and normal, physiological birth in Italy. Since then, she has set up a website covering topics relating to pregnancy, birth and breastfeeding, so as to help women make informed decisions, and she has written four other books. Also, in 2008 she launched the first international two-year year course in integrated physiology and salutogenesis (health promotion). This certified course, which is taught in German, is intended for midwives who want to learn a more positive approach to providing continuous care during pregnancy, labour and birth and who want to teach this approach to other midwives.

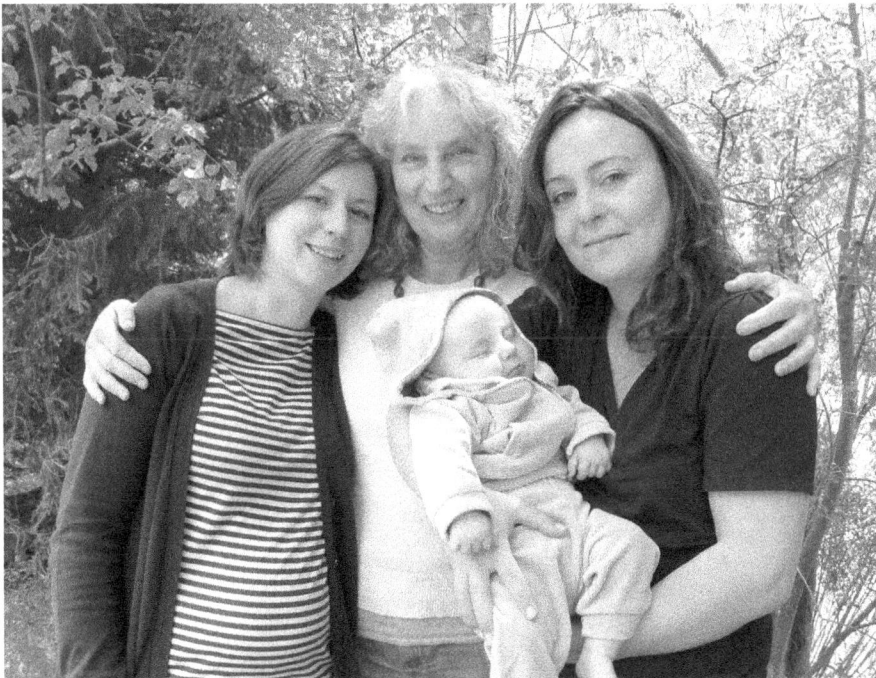

Photos © Sandro Pintus

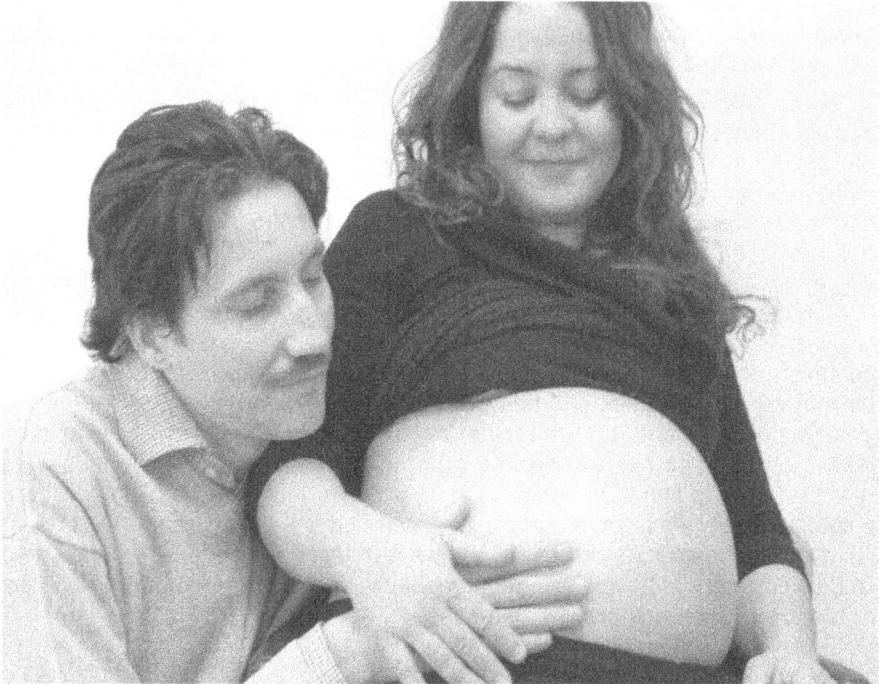

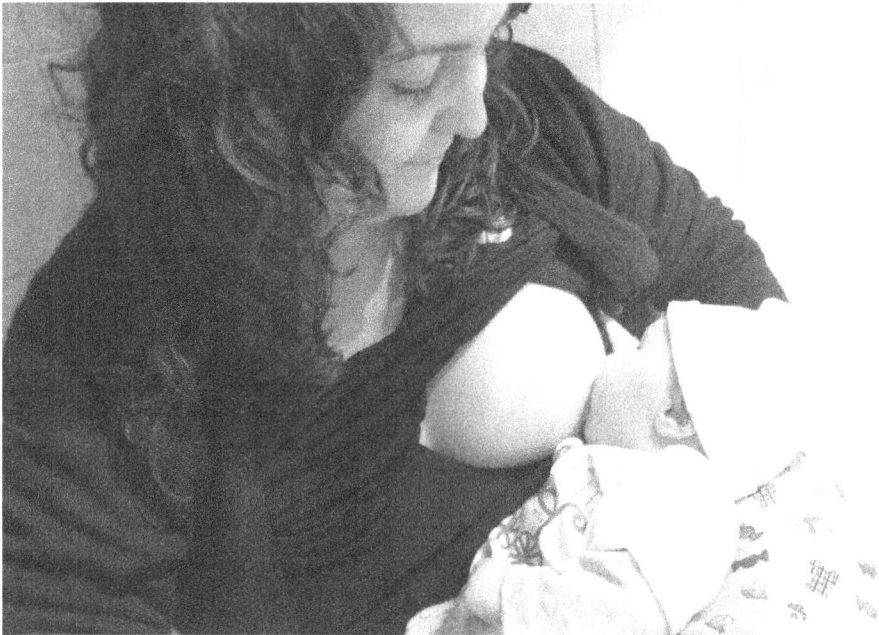

Photo © Sandro Pintus

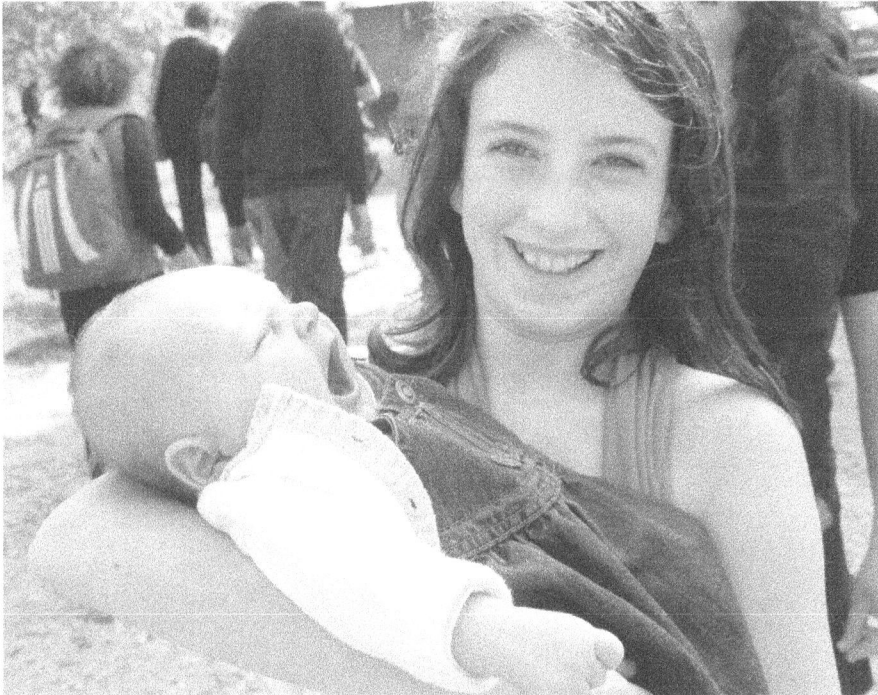

For more information or to provide feedback:

At Fresh Heart we're interested in hearing about your own experience so as to inform future books, but you may also want to have your comments published. If so, you can be named or anonymous and your comments may be used either on the website or in a book, with your permission, of course.

To contact us to tell us about your experience or for any other reason, simply click on 'Contact us' at the website below. If you're not online, write to us at:

Comments/Experience, Fresh Heart Publishing
PO Box 225, Chester le Street, DH3 9BQ

Fresh ♥ Heart

www.freshheartpublishing.co.uk

www.ingramcontent.com/pod-product-compliance
Lightning Source LLC
Chambersburg PA
CBHW080239270326
41926CB00020B/4305